teaching
AIDS

A Resource Guide on
Acquired Immune Deficiency Syndrome

REVISED EDITION

MARCIA QUACKENBUSH AND PAMELA SARGENT

Network Publications, a division of ETR Associates
Santa Cruz, CA 1988

Publisher's Note

This publication is designed to provide accurate and authoritative information in regard to the subject matter covered. It is sold with the understanding that the publishers are not engaged in rendering medical, psychological, or other professional services. If expert assistance or counseling is needed, the services of a competent professional should be sought.

Network Publications
P.O. Box 1830
Santa Cruz, CA 95061-1830

ISBN: 0-941816-41-9

Authors' Note

Every reasonable effort has been made to provide accurate information in this publication. The statements made in the curriculum are consistent with the present state of knowledge about AIDS. We do not expect substantive changes in most of this material in the near future, but cannot be responsible for inconsistencies that might arise as a result of new developments in research.

Dedication

This work is dedicated to the memory of Jon Herzstam, a long-time advocate for youth and a pioneer in planning AIDS prevention programs for young people.

Table of Contents

How This Curriculum Was Developed

In 1985, Marcia Quackenbush organized a workshop for middle and high school teachers in the San Francisco Bay area on how to teach about AIDS in their classes. Some 300 educators attended. This was one of the first trainings of its type in the country.

One of the materials distributed at the training was a curriculum on AIDS. The original curriculum contained some of the information included here. Interest in an expanded version was high, and requests for copies came in from all over the country. Teachers reviewing the original work made many helpful suggestions for improving it. Work on the new version began.

Early in 1986, ETR Associates expressed an interest in publishing an AIDS curriculum. Pamela Sargent joined the project, writing "AIDS: The Basic Unit," the teaching supplement "How AIDS Infects the Immune System," and the 10-question test. She also assisted in the planning of the science units.

We would like to thank the following people and organizations for their generous assistance in our work on this curriculum.

David Bracker
Eileen Campbell
Susan Crocker
Richard Daquioag
Kim Cox
Chuck Frutchey
Peter Goldblum
Joan Haskin

Donald Leach
JoAnn Loulan
Renetia Martin
Cheri Pies
Beth Sabin
Sylvia Villarreal
Debra Zilavy

The writing of this curriculum was supported in part by a grant from the San Francisco General Hospital AIDS Research Fund.

The list of common symptoms of AIDS (p. 12) and the explanation of the meaning of antibody test results (p. 18) are taken from two of the informational brochures distributed by the San Francisco AIDS Foundation. This material is used with permission.

"Infection Precautions for People With AIDS" (p.139) was written by Grace Lusby and Helen Schietinger, and is reprinted here with permission.

The original version of this curriculum, distributed in 1985, was written with the encouragement of the University of California San Francisco AIDS Health Project. Their moral support in the further development of this material has been greatly appreciated.

NOTES ON REVISED EDITION

This curriculum was revised during the summer of 1987, and once again the material is consistent with the present state of knowledge about AIDS. The revision consists primarily of adding additional resource material ("Teaching About Condom Use," "Instructions for Cleaning Needles," "The Issue of Abstinence," "Infection Control Guidelines for Persons with AIDS Living in the Community," "How Health Workers Can Protect Themselves from Infection on the Job," "Infection Control Guidelines for Lab Classes," "CDC Case Definition of AIDS," "CDC Classification System for HIV Infections," and Glossary), and elaborating on some issues to help clarify them. Few substantive changes were made.

In this edition, we have generally used the term "safer sex," rather than "safe sex," because it is more accurate and preferred. We speak in some cases of "transmission of the AIDS virus," rather than "transmission of AIDS," again because this is scientifically more correct. We have updated statistics. We now include oral intercourse as a "definitely unsafe" activity, where in the earlier edition we were unclear about the safety of oral sex. We no longer state that the AIDS virus must directly enter the blood stream to cause infection because it appears that in some instances, direct, prolonged and intimate contact with infected fluids, especially blood, on open cuts or mucous membranes is able to transmit the virus.

More importantly, even with the greater and more specific knowledge about AIDS in 1987, none of the standard recommendations for the prevention of infection has changed. "Safe" sexual activities remain safe, and "possibly safe" and "definitely unsafe" activities carry some risk of infection. Shared needle use continues to be a source of transmission. Casual transmission has not occurred. The epidemic grows alarmingly. Teenagers and young adults still want and deserve full, complete information about the transmission of this virus and means of preventing infection.

We wish you the best in your prevention efforts and hope the expanded and updated curriculum is useful.

USING THE CURRICULUM

Why Teach Teenagers and Young Adults About AIDS?

AIDS is a terrible disease. At present, there is no vaccine and no cure, and mortality is very high. The only way to stop the disease now is to *prevent* infection in the first place. As teachers and educators, you have the opportunity to make a significant impact on your students, to inform them about this disease and how it can be prevented, and to persuade them to follow prevention guidelines. Teaching about AIDS is an essential part of our successful battle against the spread of the disease.

AIDS cases continue to increase at a startling rate—there were over 40,000 cases reported at the time this curriculum was revised (August, 1987), and public health experts predict there will be more than 270,000 cases by the end of 1991. Each diagnosis of AIDS carries immense costs: the loss of productivity by young members of society, the significant expense of medical care, and the immeasurable costs of human suffering and loss for those diagnosed, their friends and family. What makes this doubly tragic is that this disease can be prevented.

At this point, we know for certain that AIDS is transmitted primarily through certain kinds of sexual contact and the sharing of needles in IV drug use. **Anyone, male or female, gay, bisexual or heterosexual, can contract AIDS.** Because of their sexual behavior and drug-use patterns, teenagers and young adults in the United States are certainly at risk. (AIDS has been transmitted through blood transfusions or blood products in the past, but current tests of donated blood now make the risks of such transmission extremely low.)

ADOLESCENT SEXUAL ACTIVITY

Developmentally, teenagers are in a period of their lives in which they often experiment with identities, interest, and behaviors, including sexual behaviors. The most recent national survey of the sexual practices of teenagers (the 1986 Harris Survey conducted for The Planned Parenthood Federation of America, Inc.) shows that more than half America's teenagers report having sexual intercourse by age 17. According to the 1979 surveys of two Johns Hopkins researchers, Zelnik and Kantner, some 16% of teenage women report sexual contact with four or more different partners. Eighty-five per cent of reported sexually transmitted diseases are in persons 15-30 years old. Nearly 1.2 million teenage women become pregnant each year, and at current rates, 40% of women will conceive during their teenage years. Clearly, teenagers and young adults are a sexually active population. These statistics are more startling when we consider that the same activities which caused most of these STDs and all of the pregnancies can also expose individuals to AIDS.

1

ADOLESCENT DRUG USE

Many teenagers and young adults are also likely to experiment with drugs. While national statistics on teenage IV drug use are not available, conservative estimates suggest over 200,000 high school students have used heroin; about 2 million have used other opiates; about 7 million have used stimulants; and over 3 million have used cocaine. All of these substances may be used intravenously, putting the user at risk for AIDS.

CONCLUSIONS

American teenagers throughout the country, in rural as well as urban settings, are engaging in activities which can put them at risk for AIDS.

We are fortunate that so far not many adolescents have been diagnosed with AIDS. Fewer than 1% of all U.S. cases are among teenagers. However, about 21% of total U.S. cases fall in the 20-29 year old age range. Because of the long incubation periods for AIDS— estimated now to average 5.5 years, and known to range up to at least 7 years—we know that many of these young adults were first infected with the virus as teenagers.

For the sake of their present and future health, we urge you to inform your students *now* about AIDS. They deserve accurate information about the disease. The materials in this curriculum will help you present that information effectively and thoroughly.

How To Use This Curriculum

1. **Read "Methods" and "Concepts."**
    This section summarizes the most important points to teach young people about AIDS (pp.6 and 7).

2. **Read the "Basic Information About AIDS" Section.**
    This section gives a good general background on AIDS and allows you to answer the most commonly asked questions (p.7-21).

3. **Review Other Sections of Interest.**
    Depending on your familiarity with AIDS and your experience teaching sensitive subjects, you might want to consider the suggestions in "Trouble-Shooting For Teachers: What Can Go Wrong in Teaching About AIDS?" (p. 127); "Talking About Sexuality in Classrooms" (p. 129); "Lingering Doubts About Casual Transmission" (p. 121); "Staying Updated On AIDS Information" (p. 137); "How to Teach About Condom Use" (p. 131); and "The Issue of Abstinence." (p. 125).

4. **Look Over the Teaching Plans.**
    One or more of these plans will be appropriate for your students, as presented or with some modification. The plans may also give you ideas on how to integrate information about AIDS into a curriculum you already use. Short descriptions of the plans are given on pp. 31-32, and cover sheets for each plan give more details on the material.

5. **Look Over the Teaching Materials.**
    Five worksheets and an objective test are included in this curriculum. These are optional materials which can further enhance and expand your teaching about AIDS. Descriptions are given on pp. 103-104.

6. **Teach About AIDS in Your Classes.**

Methods for Teaching
High School Students About AIDS

1.   **Present material simply.**

2.   **Be explicit and specific.** Your discussions will include information about body functions, sexual activities, IV drug use, etc. Young people need to hear very specifically what constitutes a risk activity for AIDS, as well as what exactly will protect them from infection with AIDS. Teaching will be most effective if students understand how to use condoms and where to acquire them.

3.   **If possible, present units on human sexuality before teaching about AIDS.** The absence of such a unit is no reason not to teach about AIDS, but students already exposed to the concepts of activities like anal and oral sex will be better prepared to hear information about AIDS clearly and easily.

4.   **If possible, present the basics about communicable diseases before teaching about AIDS.** Again, AIDS can certainly be taught without this information, but the fact that the AIDS virus is *not* casually transmitted makes more sense to a student who is already aware of the fact that different infectious diseases have a variety of styles of transmission.

5.   **Follow the guidelines of your school or district concerning parental consent for classes involving frank discussion of sexuality and drug use.**

Concepts for Teaching
High School Students About AIDS

There are four essential concepts all students should understand at the end of a successfully taught unit on AIDS.

1. **AIDS is a viral disease, not a gay disease.** It is not caused by a lifestyle, but by an infectious organism.

2. **AIDS is not easily transmitted.** People will not contract AIDS in normal day-to-day contact with others.

3. **Under the proper circumstances, anyone can become infected with the AIDS virus.** The AIDS virus is not influenced by a person's age, sex, or sexual orientation. Sharing IV needles or having unsafe sex with an infected person can expose anyone to AIDS.

4. **You can protect yourself against AIDS.** By not sharing IV needles (or, preferably, not using IV drugs at all), and having safe sexual contacts (or not having sex), young people can prevent exposure to AIDS.

AIDS: Basic Information

Index of Questions

USING THIS SECTION

This section will give you a good general background on AIDS and allow you to answer the most commonly asked questions. It is not necessary for you to become an expert on AIDS to teach this material effectively. If questions do arise that you are unable to answer, you can refer your students to local AIDS information sources or you can check with such groups yourself (see Worksheet 4: "Finding Answers to Questions About AIDS," p. 111).

Read the basic facts about AIDS. Pages 9 through 13 review the information recommended for an introductory lecture on AIDS, and on page 25 you will find a sample lecture.

The Most Common Questions About AIDS

DESCRIPTION/DEFINITION: *What is AIDS?*

AIDS is a disease that breaks down a part of the body's immune system, leaving a person vulnerable to a variety of unusual, life-threatening illnesses. It is caused by a virus. This virus may also infect the brain, causing a variety of neurologic problems.

The letters stand for:

Acquired - Passed from person to person. Not gotten genetically as are height and hair color.
Immune - The body's defense system, providing protection from disease.
Deficiency - Having a lack of.
Syndrome - A group of signs or symptoms which, when they occur together, mean a person has a particular disease or condition.

EPIDEMIOLOGY: *Who Gets AIDS?*

Anyone infected with the AIDS virus *might* develop AIDS.

Though gay men currently predominate in United States statistics, in some other countries virtually all cases of AIDS are among heterosexuals.

Blood for transfusions is now screened for AIDS, and blood products for hemophiliacs are treated so the AIDS virus is killed. There will be very few future infections through blood or blood products.

In 1987, the breakdown for source of infection in U.S. AIDS cases was as follows:

Population	# cases (August 1987)	% total
Gay or bisexual men	26,086	66
IV drug users	6,506	16
Hemophilia/coagulation disorder	364	1
Heterosexual contact	1,532	4
Blood transfusions	839	2
Other	1,184	3

TRANSMISSION: *How do people get AIDS?*

People do *not* get AIDS in day-to-day, casual contact with family, friends, acquaintances, workmates or the population at large -- unless that contact involves unsafe sexual encounters or the sharing of IV drugs with an infected person.

The virus that causes AIDS lives in certain body fluids, especially blood and semen. People become infected with the AIDS virus by having very intimate, very direct contact with the semen, vaginal secretions, blood (and possibly urine and feces) of someone else who is infectious. The known courses of transmission include:

1.   Sexual intercourse (vaginal, anal and oral intercourse).

2.   Shared use of needles for IV drug use. We are also concerned about the possibility of other needle use transmitting AIDS—e.g., non- professional tattooing or ear piercing among friends.

3.   Infected mothers passing the virus on to a fetus.

4.   Transfusion of blood or blood products infected with the AIDS virus (blood donations are now screened for the AIDS virus, and transfusion-related AIDS will be quite rare in the future).

Finally, a small number of health care workers who have had unusual exposure to patient blood have become infected. For example, a lab technician, because of an equipment malfunction, was splashed in the eye with copious quantities of AIDS infected blood. She has subsequently become infected herself. Instances such as these, while rare and unusual, remind health professionals to follow infection control guidelines carefully.

"I've heard that people do not get AIDS through oral sex."

There has been some controversy about transmission of the AIDS virus through oral sex. While it seems true that oral sex is not the most efficient means of transmitting the AIDS virus, a small number of people have become infected and report engaging only in oral (not vaginal or anal) intercourse. The Centers for Disease Control (CDC) is convinced by its data that oral intercourse *is* a means of transmission.

While the risk of transmission via oral sex may be lower than through vaginal or anal intercourse, the disease under consideration is severe. In the guidelines presented in this curriculum, we consider oral intercourse "definitely unsafe."

What about other "body fluids"?

The AIDS virus has been found in blood, semen, urine, vaginal secretions, spinal fluid, tears, saliva and breast milk. Of these, *only semen, vaginal secretions, blood, and possibly urine and feces are implicated in transmission.* There are also a few cases in which babies have probably contracted AIDS through infected breast milk. (Feces are considered a risk because they may also carry blood.)

People are naturally concerned about some of the other fluids—contact with tears or saliva is much more common in day-to-day life. Evidently, these other fluids do not carry a strong enough concentration of the virus to cause infection, even in the unlikely event one's blood system were to come into direct contact with them. In all reported U.S. cases so far, there is not a single case of transmission of the AIDS virus by saliva. Occasional news reports of such transmission, in the U.S. and elsewhere, have all failed to be substantiated.

So far, the AIDS virus has not been detected in sweat. Even if it is found here at a future time, sweat, like tears or saliva, is not implicated in transmission.

If you have further questions about casual transmission (via day-to-day contact), see "Lingering Doubts About Casual Transmission..." (p. 121).

SYMPTOMS: *What is it like to have AIDS?*

One of the striking qualities of this disease is the tremendous variation in how it affects different people. There are people who have been living with an AIDS diagnosis for over four years and who are still working, energetic and productive; others may die within a few days or weeks of diagnosis. Some people are fatigued or very sick throughout the course of the disease. For others, periods of health alternate with periods of illness. There are people with AIDS who are severely disabled and there are those who are in excellent physical condition. A group of San Francisco people with AIDS runs the 7-1/2 mile Bay to Breakers race every year!

At the onset of illness, most people report several of the following symptoms:

> Unexplained, persistent fatigue.
> Unexplained fever, shaking chills, or drenching night sweats lasting longer than several weeks.
> Unexplained weight loss greater than 10 pounds.
> Swollen glands (enlarged lymph nodes, usually in the neck, armpits or groin), which are otherwise unexplained and last more than two months.
> Pink to purple flat or raised blotches or bumps occurring on or under the skin, inside the mouth, nose, eyelids or rectum. Initially, they may resemble bruises but do not disappear. They are usually harder than the skin around them.
> Persistent white spots or unusual blemishes in the mouth.
> Persistent diarrhea.
> Persistent dry cough that has lasted too long to be caused by a common respiratory infection, especially if accompanied by shortness of breath.

At first glance, some of these symptoms seem much like common signs of cold, flu, etc. The key is that they are severe in nature and last over a significant period—several weeks or more—during which time usual colds or flus would have resolved. Even if symptoms are severe and long-lasting, many of these problems may actually be caused by a variety of other illnesses. AIDS CANNOT BE SELF-DIAGNOSED. Anyone concerned with symptoms should see a physician familiar with AIDS.

AIDS-RELATED COMPLEX (ARC): *What is ARC?*

The virus that causes AIDS, like many other viruses, has different effects on different people. Some people infected with the virus do not appear ill. They are asymptomatic carriers. Some may develop mild to moderate illness, while others become quite ill.

When the Centers for Disease Control (CDC) defined this viral disease, they described the most common symptoms of the disease in its most serious state. Their definition says a person has AIDS if he or she has no known underlying cause of immune system problems, but does have one of the following: (1) Kaposi's sarcoma, (2) Pneumocystis carinii pneumonia, or (3) other opportunistic infections.

People who have milder symptoms of AIDS infection, or very unusual severe symptoms, do not fit this diagnosis. They are said to have AIDS-related complex, or ARC. Some people with ARC are fairly healthy, and some are quite ill. For some, the illness progresses to death without their ever receiving an official AIDS diagnosis.

There are difficulties with this situation. For one thing, people with ARC often are not eligible for the same benefits and services as people with AIDS, though they may need such assistance. For another, the uncertainties of having ARC are many (Will I die? Will I be able to continue working? Will I recover my health?), and numerous studies have shown people with ARC experience greater anxiety than people with AIDS or those who are well. Finally, the official CDC surveillance of the disease caused by the AIDS virus only counts a small percentage of those actually affected, and the concerns of people with ARC are often neglected in health policy and research planning.

The CDC has recently (August 1987) updated its definition of AIDS. People showing signs of direct brain infection with the virus and those who have the "wasting" disease (severe and persistent loss of weight associated with AIDS virus infection) are now also considered to have AIDS. In 1986, a four-tier system of classifying all stages of AIDS infection was developed. Many people working in the AIDS field now talk more generally of people having HIV infection ("HIV" is the internationally used name for the AIDS virus—see "What Is the AIDS Virus?", p.17), rather than making many distinctions between "AIDS," "moderate ARC," "severe ARC," "mild AIDS-related symptoms," and so forth.

For a complete description of the CDC diagnostic criteria and the classifications of HIV infection, see pages 147-151.

INCUBATION: *How long is the incubation period for AIDS?*

Estimates of the incubation period for AIDS have changed as research continues and we have more experience with the disease. The most recent research suggests the average length of incubation is about five years. Many people may develop AIDS sooner than this, and in a few instances AIDS has appeared as much as seven years after exposure to the virus. Most AIDS researchers suspect that the virus could incubate for even longer periods of time.

PREVENTING AIDS: *What are the basic guidelines for AIDS prevention?*

1.   Abstain from sex; or, if you are going to engage in sexual activity, do not allow semen, vaginal secretions, blood, urine or feces of an infected person to enter your body. Use condoms for all types of intercourse.

2.   If you do not know whether or not a sexual partner is infected with AIDS, follow safer sex guidelines. Remember, you cannot tell by looking at someone whether he or she has been infected.

3.   Do not share hypodermic needles or any other needles under *any* circumstances. (It is also best not to share razors or toothbrushes with an infected person because they may expose you to minute amounts of blood.)

13

OTHER COMMON QUESTIONS

NATURAL HISTORY OF AIDS: *Does everyone infected with the AIDS virus die?*

At this point, most of the people in the U.S. infected with the AIDS virus are not ill. However, in studies of people who have been infected for some time, rates of illness are quite high. In one well-known San Francisco study, a group of men who are known to have been infected since 1978 or 1979 has been followed carefully. After seven years, about 75% of these men had AIDS, ARC or lymphadenopathy (swollen lymph glands) presumed to be related to infection with the AIDS virus. As time goes on, this number is likely to grow.

These findings are startling. If they hold true in other groups, it means that most people infected will become ill. And, while it is true that some people are only mildly ill or have episodes of illness alternating with periods of health, AIDS-related infections overall appear to be progressive in nature—that is, over time the state of health deteriorates. There is a very small number of individuals who may have recovered some of their immune functioning (their immune systems have become stronger), but most people have not done so once they become ill.

The answer to this question, then, is that we do not know if everyone infected with the AIDS virus will die. We certainly hope this is not the case. Out of respect for the thousands of people living with this disease today, it seems inappropriate to make any sort of blanket statements to this effect without better evidence than we currently have.

ADDITIONAL SAFETY: *Are there additional ways to increase one's protection from the AIDS virus in sexual intercourse?*

Spermicidal lubricants are available and can be used with condoms. Non-oxynol 9 is a substance in some of these spermicides that has been shown to kill the AIDS virus on contact. We recommend that people use a non-oxynol 9 spermicide along with a condom in vaginal and anal intercourse as "extra" insurance, in case the condom breaks. Non-oxynol 9 is *not* considered an effective preventative without a condom.

The concentration of non-oxynol 9 varies from spermicide to spermicide. To be effective, the product should carry at least 5% concentration.

Finally, any lubricant used with condoms must be *water based,* containing no fats or oils. Check labels carefully—fats and oils break down latex and cause condoms to break.

PROBLEMS WITH PREVENTION: *What keeps people from following AIDS prevention guidelines?*

There are assorted reasons people do not follow these guidelines. They may not know about AIDS prevention. They may not consider themselves at risk. Or they may know they have a risk but believe "it could never happen to me."

Condoms are an important element of safer sex practices, and many people are embarrassed or uninformed about the purchase or use of condoms. As we redefine our concepts of sexuality and increase our comfort with safer sex, we can begin to see those behaviors as complete and exciting activities.

IV drug users have traditionally had a difficult time changing behaviors. If sharing needles is the only way to get a drug to which you are addicted, it is very difficult to decide not to share. Drug users need AIDS prevention information, and we must redouble our efforts to prevent IV drug addiction and abuse in the first place.

HISTORY OF AIDS: *Why are people concerned about AIDS now? Why haven't we heard about it before?*

AIDS was not recognized or described as a disease until 1981. Tracking of AIDS only began when doctors had seen enough of it to recognize that they were faced with a serious, previously unknown disease. In 1981, 316 people in the United States had AIDS. By August 1986, over 23,000 cases were reported here. A tremendous growth in the rate of the disease has continued. This is alarming, and scientists, health professionals and the general public have all become very concerned about it.

Where did AIDS come from?

The exact origins of AIDS are not known. Either it is a new human disease which developed recently, or it is a disease that was until recently isolated in a particular geographic group of people.

The prevailing scientific opinion now is that the virus originated in Africa. A particular kind of monkey, the African green monkey, is known to carry a virus quite similar in structure to the human AIDS virus. The best scientific guess is that at some point in time, as a natural part of the process of all living organisms, there was a chance mutation of one of the simian (monkey) viruses which made it possible for the virus to cross the species barrier from monkey to human. While mutations at the cellular level are fairly common, this particular type of mutation would be very unusual.

In certain areas of Africa, the green monkey is considered a food delicacy. Possibly through ingesting some uncooked organs, or through an accidental cut while preparing a carcass, the first human was infected. The disease may have begun in this simple, quiet manner, spreading to others from this point through sexual intercourse and shared needle use.

We want to note that many African government representatives are sensitive about this view, understandably since it is often set forth in a manner that seems to blame Africa for the appearance of the virus. While scientific events are not themselves racist, observations and reporting of them may be so. It is important to remember that no one person, nation or population is responsible for the development of AIDS, and we must all share the responsibility for stopping the spread of the virus.

IMMUNOLOGY: *What happens to the immune system when someone is infected with the AIDS virus?*

The immune system is complex. In studying AIDS, medical researchers are beginning to understand more about it.

Basically, the body of a person infected with the AIDS virus may lose the ability to fight off certain infections that people with healthy immune systems can combat successfully. For instance, Pneumocystis carinii pneumonia (PCP), a common and serious infection in persons with AIDS, is caused by a one-celled organism that is all around us. Most of us have already been exposed to this organism many times throughout our lives. The body's immune system recognizes it and eliminates it without our ever becoming ill. For people with AIDS, the immune system may recognize the parasite, but the immune response is damaged so the body is unable to fight the infection, and the person becomes ill. The kinds of diseases that infect a person with this kind of immune problem are called "opportunistic infections." (For a more in-depth explanation of how AIDS infects the immune system, see Plan 6: "The AIDS Virus" [p. 77]. For a simple explanation appropriate for classes, with diagrams, see Supplement: "How the AIDS Virus Infects the Immune System" [p. 99].)

RANGE OF INFECTIONS: *What are the illnesses that affect people with AIDS?*

The manifestations of AIDS can vary widely from person to person. The range of infections seen in AIDS is quite broad, with people being affected by fungal, bacterial, protozoal and viral diseases as well as some cancers. The two most common AIDS diseases are Kaposi's sarcoma and Pneumocystis carinii pneumonia. Kaposi's sarcoma (KS) is a cancer of the cells that line certain small blood vessels. People with KS develop purple lesions, which may appear on the skin where they can be seen or internally where they cannot be seen. In time, the number of lesions will usually increase and they may grow in size. As the disease progresses, complications may develop because of the number and size of lesions.

Pneumocystis carinii pneumonia (PCP) is the most common opportunistic infection seen in people with AIDS. It is caused by a protozoan, a microscopic organism. People with PCP usually become quite ill at the time of diagnosis, with fatigue, weight loss, fevers, dry cough and difficulty breathing. Often PCP requires hospitalization. This disease can be treated. As with other AIDS-related diseases, successful treatment of PCP does not cure the underlying immune problems. In time a person may again be affected by PCP or other opportunistic infections.

Other infections seen in AIDS include toxoplasmosis and cryptosporidium, also caused by protozoans; candida and cryptococcus, caused by fungi; cytomegalovirus (CMV) and herpes, caused by viruses (herpes infections in people with AIDS are *quite* severe and atypical; the usual genital or oral herpes infections are *not* indicative of AIDS); and a bacterial disease called mycobacterium avium intracellularis. (For a more in-depth description of AIDS- related diseases, see Plan 6: "The AIDS Virus" [p. 77].)

VIROLOGY: *What is the AIDS virus?*

There continues to be some debate about the AIDS virus including what group of viruses it belongs to and whether it is the sole cause of AIDS or if there are other causes as well. These issues are currently under research. What is known is that the AIDS virus is one of a special kind of viruses called "retroviruses." When a person is infected, the virus takes over certain cells in the immune system, destroying the cells' disease-fighting capabilities. The virus then uses the reproductive mechanisms of the cell to reproduce more virus. It has been difficult to control retroviruses.

The AIDS virus has been given a variety of names by different researchers, including HTLV-3, LAV, and ARV. In 1986, an international panel suggested it be called HIV—"Human Immunodeficiency Virus." This is the name used commonly now.

The AIDS virus is also a fragile virus, which does not live long or well outside the human body. It is easily killed with a 1:10 solution of bleach and water, and can be washed from hands or skin with regular soaps.

There have been reports of AIDS virus surviving outside the body for periods of several days. In these studies, massive concentrations of virus were used. The actual concentration of the virus in blood or semen is *many* magnitudes less, so in any natural biological state the virus will *not* survive outside the human body for more than a few hours at most.

VACCINE: *When will there be a vaccine for AIDS?*

To date, a successful vaccine has never been developed for a human retrovirus, which makes finding an AIDS vaccine one of the greatest challenges for medical science so far. There is still no guarantee that a vaccine for AIDS can be produced, but recent developments are promising. Guesses for when a vaccine will appear run anywhere from two to ten years, and some experts believe it will never happen.

Once and if a vaccine is developed, it will need to be tested carefully for several years before it is used widely. The only course for preventing AIDS at present is to practice the AIDS prevention guidelines (p. 13).

AIDS ANTIBODY TESTING: *What is the AIDS antibody test?*

The AIDS antibody test is an inexpensive screening test that was developed to make certain blood donated for transfusions did not carry the AIDS virus. There are actually three different tests currently being used to check for AIDS antibodies, each using a different method. The most common type is an ELISA ("ELISA" refers to the method of assay used). The ELISA tells, fairly simply and quite inexpensively, whether a blood specimen has been infected with the AIDS virus. It is a practical way to screen blood donations and, because it is now universally applied in U.S. blood banks, it has made the blood supply very safe. We will probably see very few future cases of AIDS passed through transfusions (though people transfused before 1985 may still be at risk because of the incubation period of the disease; see p. 13 for more information). The test is usually used to test semen donors for insemination, and it is recommended for organ donors to protect recipients of organ transplants.

Some individuals have taken the antibody test to determine whether or not they have been infected with the AIDS virus. If the antibody is *absent*, the test is *negative* and it means *one* of the following is true:

1.   The person has not been infected with the virus.

OR

2.   The person has had contact with the AIDS virus but has not become infected and therefore has not produced antibodies. However, repeated exposure to the AIDS virus would increase the likelihood that the person will become infected.

OR

3.   The person has been infected by the virus but has not yet produced antibodies. Research indicates most people will produce antibodies within 2-12 weeks after infection. Some people will not produce antibodies for six months or more. A very small number of people will never produce antibodies.

If the test shows that the antibody is *present*, the test is *positive*, and it means *all* of the following are true:

1.   The person's blood sample has been tested and the test indicates antibodies to the virus are present.

AND

2.   The person has been infected with the AIDS virus and antibodies have been produced.

AND

3.   Researchers have shown that most people with AIDS antibodies have active virus in their bodies. Therefore, a person with a positive test must assume he or she is capable of passing the virus on to others under the correct circumstances for transmission (see "Transmission," p.10).

The test is quite accurate, but like other medical tests there will be some false negatives (a person *does* have antibody, but tests negative) and false positives (a person *does not* have antibody but tests positive).

The ELISA test was developed to screen blood donations. The blood banks naturally wanted to be very careful to pull out any blood infected with the AIDS virus, so this test is more likely to err on the side of false positives (that is, it would be better to pull out non-infected blood, losing a few units of blood that were actually safe), than false negatives (allowing blood that *was* infected to be used for transfusions). To correct for this error of the test, responsible labs will usually screen blood first with the ELISA, because it is the easiest and most inexpensive test available. If the sample tests positive, they will test it two more times with the ELISA and, if both of these tests are positive, the sample will be checked again with one of the other types of tests. When these procedures are followed, results are accurate well over 99% of the time.

Unfortunately, some labs, especially some private-for-profit operations, have not been as careful as this. They will report results based on a single ELISA screening. Under these circumstances, the error rate is much higher. People wanting to take the test might want to ask about lab procedures before they do so.

Many people misunderstand the antibody test and believe it is a "test for AIDS." It will not tell whether a person has AIDS or AIDS-related complex (ARC), or whether a person will or will not develop AIDS or ARC.

If a person wants to take the AIDS antibody test, we recommend having the test performed where anonymity is guaranteed if possible. Anonymous testing means your name and test results are not recorded together anywhere, nor is there any record of your taking the test. A mention of the test in medical records, even if the results are negative, might complicate future efforts to acquire health insurance. In some states a positive result could lead to legal problems.

HETEROSEXUAL TRANSMISSION: *What is the risk of heterosexuals contracting AIDS?*

Anyone can contract AIDS if he or she is exposed to the virus through unsafe sex or the sharing of IV needles.

Most experts do not consider it likely that AIDS will spread as rapidly among heterosexuals as it has with gay men because heterosexuals generally have fewer sexual partners. A small number of well-informed researchers, however, feel heterosexuals should be more alerted to AIDS risks than they have been. AIDS can be spread by vaginal intercourse, and there are cases of male-to-female and female-to-male transmission. Those at highest risk are people with multiple sexual partners in areas where the disease is already widespread. In some countries, virtually all of those affected with AIDS are heterosexuals.

For most U.S. heterosexuals, the risk of contracting AIDS today is small. The judicious use of safer sex practices (along with not sharing IV needles) can keep the risk small in the future.

LESBIAN TRANSMISSION: *Can lesbians get AIDS?*

A few cases have now been reported of sexual transmission of the AIDS virus between lesbians. We recommend that lesbians consider partners' sexual histories and any past IV drug use. If there is a possibility of risk, they should practice safer sex. Like everyone else, lesbians are also susceptible to AIDS infection through IV drug use or unsafe sexual contact with infected men.

PREGNANCY: *How are people to plan pregnancies if the AIDS virus can be transmitted by semen?*

If two people wish to consider pregnancy and they know confidently that neither has a past risk of exposure to AIDS, they can simply proceed with their plans.

In assessing risk, one must consider (1) history of IV drug use; (2) personal sexual history; (3) the sexual and drug use histories of any past sexual partners; and (4) any history of blood or blood product transfusion. It is difficult to know confidently about the history of past partners, and one would want to consider one's experience since 1978.

If there is some doubt about the possibility of exposure to AIDS, couples might consider taking the AIDS antibody test (explained on p. 18). If one or both partners have been exposed to the AIDS virus, we recommend postponing pregnancy until we have a way to prevent transmission of the virus to partners or a fetus. Donors providing semen for insemination should be tested for AIDS antibodies.

INSECT BITES: *Can people get AIDS from insect bites?*

A good amount of study has been focused on this subject, and most of the scientific community is well-convinced that this is not a mode of transmission. In a recent study, however, some mosquitoes fed AIDS-infected blood were found to be carrying virus as much as two days afterwards. Naturally, this information causes concern. It is important to remember, however, that while mosquitoes do withdraw blood from people, they do not exchange blood between people.

A careful look at epidemiology makes this clearer. Malaria is a widespread disease in Africa that *is* spread by mosquitoes. The insects first ingest the parasite which causes malaria by feeding on an infected person, then transmit the parasite through their saliva to another person several days later. People of all ages are infected, including children and elders who may not be sexually active. AIDS, on the other hand, is a disease spread by shared needle use and intimate sexual contact, and the people in both Africa and the U.S. who are infected or diagnosed with AIDS fall into very specific categories of risk. They do not represent the more general population of individuals bitten by mosquitoes.

A community in Florida, Belle Glade, has a very high incidence of AIDS. Many of the residents are farm workers, who might receive hundreds of mosquito bites in a day. Studies there specifically sought to determine whether mosquitoes were implicated in transmission of AIDS. The studies showed that residents of Belle Glade infected or diagnosed with AIDS have the same kinds of risks other people have had—sharing needles in IV drug use, or sexual contact with persons at risk (primarily heterosexual contact in these cases). Those with high incidences of mosquito bites without other risk factors did *not* become infected.

SCHOOLS: *What is the likelihood of a middle or high school student with the AIDS virus passing it on to other students (or teachers) in my school?*

Remember the means of AIDS transmission: a person must have very intimate, very direct contact with the semen, vaginal secretions, blood, urine or feces of an infected person. A student is *very* unlikely to have interactions on a school campus that would allow this transmission to occur. Unless the student is having sex with others, or sharing IV needles, there just is not much chance of AIDS being transmitted.

People with AIDS or ARC need to be supported in living the most productive lives possible. School is the productive work of teenagers. Students with AIDS/ARC would do best being enrolled in normal classes unless their illness was too severe to allow them to participate.

We note also that guidelines issued by the Centers for Disease Control as well as The American Academy of Pediatrics recommend that students with AIDS/ARC continue attending regular school classes.

CASUAL TRANSMISSION: *I'm not convinced that AIDS can't be transmitted casually. There's too much we don't know about the disease.*

For a fuller discussion of this issue, see "Lingering Doubts About Casual Transmission," p. 121.

Safe and Unsafe Sexual Activities

Definitely safe:
(no exchange of semen, vaginal secretions, blood, urine or feces)

Touching, hugging, massage
Masturbation, alone or with a partner
Rubbing bodies together
Talking about sex, verbal fantasies
Social kissing (dry)
Kissing or licking the body (clean skin; no oral contact with genitals or any open sores)

Probably safe:
(most likely there would be no exchange of semen, vaginal secretions, blood, urine or feces)

Vaginal intercourse with a condom (as long as the condom is used properly and does not break)
Oral intercourse with a condom or latex barrier over the genitals (proper use, no breakage)
Anal intercourse with a condom (proper use, no breakage)
French kissing (wet) (unless the kiss is very hard and draws blood, or either partner has open sores or infection in or around mouth)

Definitely unsafe:
(almost certain dangerous exchange of semen, vaginal secretions, blood, urine or feces)

Vaginal intercourse without a condom
Oral intercourse without a condom or latex barrier
Anal intercourse without a condom
Sharing objects inserted into anus or vagina
Any activity that allows blood-to-blood contact

Sample Lecture

AIDS stands for Acquired Immune Deficiency Syndrome. It's a disease that breaks down a part of the body's immune system so the person with AIDS can get a variety of unusual, life-threatening illnesses that healthy people don't get. It's a very serious disease.

You may have heard that AIDS is a disease gay men get. That's true, but other people get it as well. Women and children, babies, IV drug users, heterosexuals, even some teenagers have gotten AIDS. In the United States today, most of the people with AIDS *are* gay or bisexual men. An increasing number of heterosexuals are being affected too. In some countries, almost all cases of AIDS are among heterosexuals.

AIDS is caused by a virus. *Anyone* infected with that virus can become ill, regardless of age, sex, race, sexual orientation, or anything else.

The AIDS virus, just like many other viruses, can cause a wide range of symptoms. There are basically three ways people might show infection with the AIDS virus:

1.   Many people infected with the virus look and feel perfectly healthy. Such people can pass the virus on to others. They are called "asymptomatic carriers," that is, carriers without symptoms of the disease.

2.   Other people develop symptoms related to AIDS, but do not have one of the diseases that medical researchers use to diagnose AIDS. These people are said to have AIDS related complex (ARC). They can be fairly healthy or quite sick. Some people with ARC may become so ill they die without ever being diagnosed with AIDS.

3.   Finally, some people infected with the virus develop full-blown AIDS. This is usually the most serious form of the disease. Over half the people diagnosed with AIDS so far have died, and very few have survived five years.

Because many people are healthy carriers of AIDS and do not know they are infectious, it has been hard to stop the spread of the disease. The AIDS virus also has a long incubation period—it can take quite a while between the time a person is first infected and the time he or she actually gets sick. With AIDS, this might take anywhere from several weeks to seven years or more.

Fortunately, AIDS is a *difficult* disease to get. Let me tell you some of the things you can

25

do that will *not* expose you to the AIDS virus. You *cannot* get AIDS by touching or hugging someone, sharing food or drinks, riding buses. You *cannot* get it from toilet seats or sinks or swimming pools or hot tubs. You *cannot* get it from drinking fountains. You *cannot* get it by sharing telephones, paper or pencils. You *cannot* get it from someone coughing or sneezing on you. You *cannot* get it from donating blood.

People get AIDS by having very intimate, very direct contact with the semen, vaginal secretions, blood, urine or feces of someone else infected with the virus. Here are some ways that might happen:

1. The AIDS virus can be passed between sexual partners engaging in either vaginal, anal, or oral intercourse.

2. The AIDS virus can enter the blood stream directly when IV drug users share needles. AIDS may be transmitted by people sharing needles for tattooing or ear-piercing without sterilizing them properly.

3. In the past, some people have gotten AIDS from blood transfusions, or from special blood products for people with diseases like hemophilia. Now, blood donations are screened and tested, so the blood supply is quite safe. The medicines for people with hemophilia are pasteurized (heat-treated) to destroy the virus.

4. Women infected with the AIDS virus can pass the virus to newborn children. The children are infected before birth, when they share the mother's blood system.

These are the ways we know that the AIDS virus is transmitted. We know it is not spread by casual contact. Even transmission by saliva (kissing, for example), sweat or tears, doesn't happen. In all the cases reported in the United States (more than 40,000 as of August 1987), we have never seen such transmission. You might occasionally read about cases where this is claimed to have happened, but on closer investigation, none of these claims has been true.

Since you can see now that AIDS is not easy to get, and since you know the ways people *can* get it, what can people do to make sure they don't get it?

Two simple rules:

1. Think carefully about whether you want to have sex with someone else. Abstinence is 100% effective in preventing the sexual transmission of AIDS.

    If you *do* decide to have sex, don't take any body fluids directly into your body during any kind of sexual intercourse. Use condoms (rubbers) - they are able to stop the AIDS virus when used correctly.

2. Don't share needles for IV drugs or tattoos *ever.*

Remember that you cannot tell just by looking at someone whether he or she has been exposed to the virus. Some people infected with AIDS look and feel very healthy. Your best bet is to follow these two prevention guidelines all the time.

TEACHING PLANS

Introduction to Teaching Plans

These seven teaching plans present different approaches to teaching AIDS in the classroom. Each plan covers the important basic information about AIDS: (1) it is not casually transmitted; (2) under certain circumstances *anyone* can be infected, regardless of sexual orientation or gender; and (3) AIDS can be prevented. Most plans are designed so they can be taught in a single-session class or expanded to fill two or three sessions. It is our belief that AIDS is an important and complex enough issue that it deserves two or three sessions, but we acknowledge that not all teachers have the luxury of setting aside this amount of time for a new curriculum topic.

1. **The Basic AIDS Unit: A One-Class Module**

    This unit is especially useful for broad-scale teaching of AIDS, throughout an entire school or district, for instance.

2. **Public Response to AIDS**
    (Social Studies, Psychology, Current Events)

    This unit examines the range of responses to the AIDS epidemic.

3. **Civil Rights Issues and AIDS**
    (Civics, Social Studies, History, Ethics)

    This unit examines the important relationships between civil liberties and public welfare, using AIDS as a current and relevant example.

4. **Epidemics and AIDS**
    (History, Social Studies, Science)

    This unit presents basic AIDS information in the context of other epidemics through history.

5. **STDs and AIDS**
    (Family Life Education, Sex Education, Health Education)

    These materials can be integrated into any already-existing unit on STDs, such as might be offered in a family life, sex education or health education class.

6.   **The AIDS Virus**
     (Biology, Physiology, Immunology, General Science)

     This unit presents basic information about the AIDS virus: how it replicates, how it affects the immune system, and what some of the diseases are that strike people with AIDS.

7.   **Pursuing a Medical Mystery: The Story of AIDS**
     (Biology, Physiology, General Science)

     The practice of epidemiology is described using AIDS as a current and relevant example.

     Supplement: How AIDS Infects the Immune System

     A simple explanation of how AIDS infects the immune system, with accompanying diagrams.

Plan 1: AIDS—The Basic Unit

Target:
General classes. Broad-scale teaching.

Purpose:
To communicate risk information for AIDS, risk-reduction guidelines, and clarify that the AIDS virus is not spread by casual contact.

Objectives:
1. Students will know basic information about AIDS transmission.
2. Students will know general risk-reduction guidelines for AIDS.

Format:
1. Lecture/discussion.
2. Written exercises.
3. Objective exam.

Materials:
1. Lecture aids (Diagrams 1-A through 1-E).

2. Any of the worksheets can be used in this unit. Worksheet 1 and Worksheet 4 are especially recommended.

3. Test.

Time:
50 minutes (one full class period).
Optional written exercises (Worksheets 2-6) offer further opportunity for follow-up at a later class session if desired.

Utilization:
Following the outlines, present the class with a series of questions, lecture and discussions to present basic information about AIDS and impress upon students the relevance of this information.

NOTE: "AIDS—The Basic Unit" presents only the most essential information teenagers and young adults need to have about AIDS. We believe AIDS is a very complex and important issue that deserves in-depth attention. We encourage and recommend, therefore, that this basic unit be expanded upon whenever possible, using portions of other plans in this curriculum, worksheets, or other appropriate materials.

PLAN 1: AIDS --THE BASIC UNIT

Method: Follow the outlines below. There are questions and lecture material included. Vignettes ("Samuel and Shari" and "Toshi's Story") provide discussion opportunities.

NOTE: It is fairly common, after hearing about safer sex practices, that students will have questions about planning pregnancies. This information is reviewed in "Basic Information About AIDS," pages 7-21.

SECTION I: INTRODUCTION

A.   Tell students you will be discussing the disease AIDS in class today.

B.   (Optional) Have students spend a few minutes filling out Worksheet 1: "Personal Opinions About AIDS." Remind them there are no right or wrong answers.

SECTION II: ASSESSING STUDENTS' KNOWLEDGE ABOUT AIDS

A.   What do you already know about AIDS? What kinds of rumors or jokes do you hear in school or from your friends?

(This question provides a baseline for understanding students' knowledge about AIDS and what areas will need focus in the class. For example, students reporting rumors that AIDS can be caught by sitting next to someone on a bus show a common misconception about casual contagion that can be addressed with education on AIDS transmission.)

B.   What have you heard about how AIDS is spread? You can mention facts, myths, or things you are not sure about.

(You could write some of these answers on the board.)

SECTION III: BASIC INFORMATION ABOUT AIDS

A.   Present the sample lecture, pages 25-27, or your own lecture, including the following:

What is AIDS?
Who gets AIDS?
How do people get AIDS?

What is it like to have AIDS?
What is ARC?
How long is the incubation period for AIDS?
What are the basic guidelines for AIDS prevention?
    (List of safe and unsafe sexual activities - p. 23)

SECTION IV: MAKING THE INFORMATION RELEVANT

A.   What has all this got to do with you and me? Is there any way you can see your life being influenced by the AIDS epidemic?

B.   Vignette: Samuel and Shari

(Diagrams 1-A through 1-E, p. 40 through p.42, can be used as teaching aids for this vignette.)

A young man named Samuel goes to a party one night, and his buddies urge him to shoot some IV drugs. He has never used drugs before, but decides he will try it just once. His friends show him what to do. Samuel doesn't know it, but one of the other people he is "shooting" with has been infected with the AIDS virus. Samuel becomes infected too. (Diagram 1-A.)

Samuel's girlfriend Shari has sex with Samuel. She becomes infected too (Diagram 1-B), though neither of them knows this.

Several months later, Samuel and Shari break up. Samuel becomes sexually involved with Marjorie, and he continues to use IV drugs on occasion. Shari starts going steady with Victor and in time they develop a sexual relationship too. Marjorie and Victor become infected with the virus, as do some people Samuel has been using drugs with (Diagram 1-C).

As each of these individuals continues, over time, to have further IV drug contacts or unsafe sex with others, the virus continues to spread (Diagram 1-D).

It is now three years since Samuel went to the party where he was infected. He left town six months ago, and no one has seen him since. You and I come into the picture here, where we might become involved with one of these people who has had direct or indirect contact with Samuel, Shari, Marjorie or Victor (Diagram 1-E). Perhaps this person only experimented with sex or drugs once. Because the AIDS infection can incubate for several years, no one even suspects him or herself to be at risk. Everyone in this picture looks and feels very healthy.

What could you do if you wanted to be sure to protect yourself from infection with the AIDS virus?

    1.   Don't use drugs. Don't share needles.

    2.   Don't have sex.

3.   Have safer sex—use condoms, don't exchange semen, vaginal secretions, blood, urine, feces during sex.

SECTION V: PROBLEM SOLVING

A.   About 50% of high school students nationally report being sexually active. What about this school—do you think that number is higher or lower?

B.   What do students in this school need to know about AIDS?

C.   What are some reasons people might put themselves at risk for infection by the AIDS virus?

1.   People might not know about AIDS.

2.   People might not know how AIDS is transmitted, so they might not know if they are putting themselves at risk.

3.   Sexual risks—a person:

a.   Might not know about safer sex, or might not understand exactly what it is.

b.   Might know about safer sex but be embarrassed to bring it up with a partner.

c.   Might be embarrassed about buying condoms, might not know where to get them, or might not be able to afford them.

d.   Might not like safer sex (believing, for example, that condoms decrease sensation, or that a safer activity like masturbation is not "real" sex).

e.   Might have a partner who does not want to practice safer sex.

f.   Others?

4.   Needle use:

a.   An IV drug user probably does not have clean needles available.

b.   A needle user may not know how to clean a needle he or she does have.

c.   An addict may need a drug so badly that concerns about AIDS are not important at the time.

d.   A person sharing needles for steroids, vitamin injections, tattooing, ear piercing, may not think of these activities as AIDS risks.

    e.   Others?

D. How can we help change people's beliefs and behaviors about safer sex?

    1.   Encourage abstinence. (Would this work in this school? Why or why not?)

    2.   Educate everyone about safer sex.

        a.   Let everyone know what safer sex is.

        b.   Educate people about condom use, including how and where to get condoms, how to use them, how to talk about condom use with partners.

        c.   Educate about how to make safer sex satisfying.

    3.   Show people on TV or in movies practicing abstinence or safer sex.

    4.   Others?

SECTION VI: TOSHI'S STORY

Toshi, a man in his early twenties, is home alone while his wife and son are out of town. He is invited to a party by some friends. At this party, some of his friends are using IV drugs. A friend keeps asking him if he wants to try the drug. Toshi at first says no, but after having a few beers, he thinks to himself, "Why not?" Toshi doesn't even know what drug he is trying.

Many months later, Toshi calls his friends to see how they are. He finds out one of the people he shared drugs with at the party has since died of AIDS. Frightened, he takes a test for the AIDS antibody. His result is positive. A counselor at the testing site tells him that this means he has been infected with the AIDS virus. It does not necessarily mean he will get AIDS, but he certainly can pass the virus on to others. This means that he could pass an AIDS infection to his wife if he has unsafe sex with her.

A. What might some of Toshi's concerns be?

    1.   He might get sick.

    2.   He might have passed the virus to his wife, or he might pass it to her in the future.

    3.   He feels he should tell his wife.

    4.   He is afraid others will find out.

5.   He is concerned for his child's health.

6.   Others?

(Toshi's concerns for his son offer an excellent opportunity to reinforce that AIDS is not casually transmitted. Because Toshi was not infected with the AIDS virus until after his son was born, the boy is not at risk to develop AIDS.)

B.   How might Toshi feel about telling his wife?

1.   Fine—depending on the relationship.
2.   Afraid.
3.   Guilty.
4.   Others?

C.   Why might Toshi be afraid of telling his wife?

1.   She might leave him.
2.   She might tell other people.
3.   She might refuse to let him see his child.
4.   She might be very angry or hurt.
5.   Others?

D.   What do you think about what Toshi did?

E.   Do you think he did anything wrong?

F.   What do you think he should do now?

G.   Do you think Toshi's experience could happen to anyone you know? Do you think anyone you know could ever be exposed to AIDS?

SECTION VII: CONCLUSIONS

A.   If students filled out Worksheet 1, have them look, over their answers on the worksheet, and ask the following questions:

1.   Would you change any of your original answers now? If you would, mark those changes in.

2.   Turn over your sheet and write down the most important thing you learned today.

B.   Give test (p. 117) to measure student comprehension. If time is short, the test can be given during the next class session.

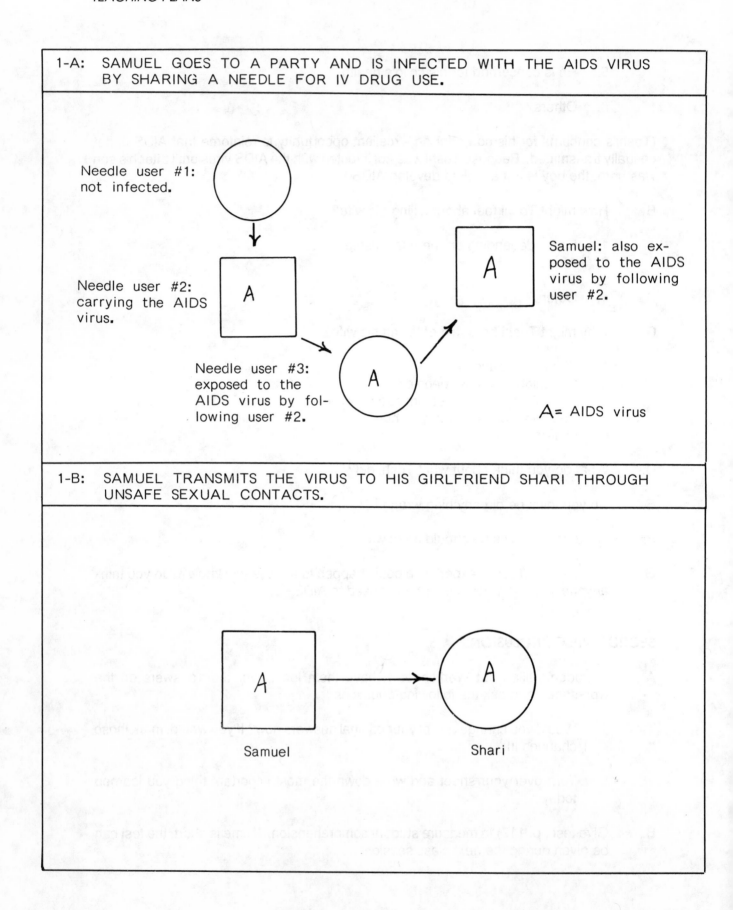

1-A: SAMUEL GOES TO A PARTY AND IS INFECTED WITH THE AIDS VIRUS BY SHARING A NEEDLE FOR IV DRUG USE.

Needle user #1: not infected.

Needle user #2: carrying the AIDS virus.

Needle user #3: exposed to the AIDS virus by following user #2.

Samuel: also exposed to the AIDS virus by following user #2.

A = AIDS virus

1-B: SAMUEL TRANSMITS THE VIRUS TO HIS GIRLFRIEND SHARI THROUGH UNSAFE SEXUAL CONTACTS.

Samuel

Shari

1-C: SAMUEL AND SHARI BREAK UP. SAMUEL BECOMES SEXUALLY IN-VOLVED WITH MARJORIE. SHARI BECOMES SEXUALLY INVOLVED WITH VICTOR. SAMUEL SHARES NEEDLES WITH OTHERS.

People who have shared IV needles with Samuel.

Marjorie   Samuel

Shari   Victor

1-D: OVER TIME, EACH OF THESE INDIVIDUALS CONTINUES TO HAVE SEXUAL OR IV NEEDLE CONTACT WITH OTHERS. THE VIRUS CON-TINUES TO SPREAD.

Sexual and drug use partners of infected IV drug users.

IV drug users infected by Samuel.

Marjorie   Samuel

Shari   Victor

41

1-E: WHAT CAN YOU DO TO PROTECT YOURSELF IF <u>YOU</u> COME INTO THE PICTURE?

Marjorie

Shari

Victor

YOU

Plan 2: Public Response to AIDS

Target:

Social studies, psychology, current events.
Classes in which discussions might commonly include personal reflection and analytic thinking about others.

Purpose:

1. To assist students in assessing public attitudes toward people with AIDS.

2. To allow students to explore their own personal response to the epidemic.

3. To communicate risk information for AIDS, risk-reduction guidelines, and clarify that the AIDS virus is not spread by casual contact.

Objectives:

1. Students will know basic information about AIDS transmission.
2. Students will know general risk-reduction guidelines for AIDS.

Format:

1. Lecture/discussion.
2. Written exercises (optional).
3. Test (optional).

Materials:

1. Worksheets 1, 2 or 3 (optional).
2. Test (optional).

Time:

1-3 full class sessions (at teacher's discretion).

Utilization:

Present a short lecture on AIDS. Select one or more of the discussion sections for the class. Facilitate the discussion, using the suggested questions as guidelines.

PLAN 2: PUBLIC RESPONSE TO AIDS

Method: Present the "Basic Information About AIDS" lecture. Then select one or more of the following sections for discussion.

BASIC INFORMATION ABOUT AIDS

Present the sample lecture, page 25, or your own lecture, including the following:

> What is AIDS?
> Who gets AIDS?
> How do people get AIDS?
> What is it like to have AIDS?
> What is ARC?
> How long is the incubation period for AIDS?
> What are the basic guidelines for AIDS prevention?
> (List of safe and unsafe sexual activities—p. 23)

SECTION I: GENERAL DISCUSSION ON AIDS

A. What are some responses people have had to AIDS?
    What are the responses of people you know?
    What are the responses of people you have heard of or read about?
    What are your own responses to AIDS?

Possible answers:

1. Helping out: donating time, money, services, etc., to people with AIDS, to education programs, to research.

2. Learning more about the disease. Staying informed.

3. Educating others about AIDS.

4. Supporting AIDS prevention. Practicing safer sex, not sharing needles.

5. Being afraid of getting AIDS.

6. Telling jokes about AIDS.

7. Blaming people with AIDS for getting sick.

8. Discriminating against people with AIDS, or against gay men, in the mistaken belief that AIDS is casually transmitted.

    a. Firing people from jobs.
    b. Evicting people from homes.
    c. Not letting a person with AIDS ride a bus.
    d. Others?

9. Trying to set up legal means to restrict or protect people with AIDS or those believed to be at risk.

B. Why are some people afraid of getting AIDS?

Possible answers:

1. Some people are truly at risk, because of sexual or drug practices, or for other reasons. Their fears may be well-founded.

2. Some people are not actually at risk for the disease, but misunderstand they might get AIDS in situations where they cannot get it (such as public pools, restaurants, schools, etc.) Their fears are unfounded.

C. All of a sudden, we seem to be hearing a lot about AIDS. There are other serious diseases around, and some are transmitted more easily than AIDS. Why do people seem more concerned about AIDS, and why is everyone talking about it now?

NOTE: An example of a serious and more easily transmitted disease is Hepatitis-B. This disease, like AIDS, is blood borne, and is most often passed through sexual contact or the sharing of needles in IV drug use. It takes *much* less contact with the Hepatitis-B virus to become infected with the disease, and it can be fatal if not properly treated.

Possible answers:

1. AIDS is a very serious disease that has received a lot of attention. Other diseases might be less serious, or may have received less attention.

2. AIDS is a *new* epidemic, and it is happening *now*. The incidence is increasing. Many other diseases have stable incidences, or an incidence rate that is increasing more slowly than that of AIDS.

3. People misunderstand or are misinformed about transmission, and believe that AIDS can be transmitted in a casual way, or that it is easy to get AIDS.

NOTE: We know that some viruses and other disease-causing organisms are passed through sneezes, sharing cups, dirty hands, etc. It may be hard for some people to adjust their understanding of diseases, distinguishing this more-casually-transmitted type of virus from the very different, difficult-to- transmit AIDS virus. This is especially likely because AIDS is such a serious disease.

    4.   People associate AIDS with death and disability, and these are frightening.

    5.   Some people have a fear of association: "If you get AIDS, people will think you're gay."

    6.   Some people are frightened of homosexuality (or IV drug use) and in their minds cannot separate AIDS from homosexuals (or IV drug users).

    7.   AIDS has some important ramifications for sexual practices. Even for people who are not in a high risk group, concerns about contracting AIDS may lead them to change their styles of sexual activity.

    8.   Others?

SECTION II: "AIDS HYSTERIA"

There are people who have labeled some responses to AIDS as "hysterical"— overemotional reactions not based in fact. Other people might call these behaviors reasonable. What do you think about the following situations?

Case 1: In New York City, at the beginning of the 1985 school year, parents of some 18,000 students refused to allow their children to attend public schools because they had heard a child with AIDS would be attending one of the district's schools.

A.   Was this a "hysterical" reaction, or a reasonable one? Why?

B.   Was there an actual risk of these children contracting AIDS from another student?

NOTE: There is no risk unless the students are engaging in a risk activity in school (e.g., having unsafe sex or sharing needles). This is obviously quite unlikely. Sharing of bathrooms, cafeterias, school materials, etc., is *not* a risk. Other scenarios—bites, fights, accidents—are not likely to transmit the virus. However, an elementary age or older student with behavioral problems leading to biting, fighting or accidents, who *was* infected with the AIDS virus, probably should *not* be attending school.

In several studies of families where one child was affected with AIDS, sibling-to-sibling transmission has never been discovered. If AIDS is not transmitted in the more intimate setting of family relationships, it is not likely to be transmitted in the schools.

C.   What would you say to a parent who refused to allow his or her child to attend school under these circumstances?

Case 2: Jack worked in a large office as a word-processor. He was diagnosed with AIDS and was placed on disability. After his initial period of illness, he was feeling well and able to return to work. When he contacted his company about his plans to return, they informed him he was not to come back to the office. His disability benefits continued, but Jack wanted to work again. His boss, Larry, said he made the decision because he wanted to protect the welfare of others in the office who used the same drinking fountain, kitchen, telephones, supplies, and restroom as Jack.

A.   Was Jack being reasonable in expecting to return to work?

B.   Were Larry's concerns about the welfare of the other workers in the office legitimate?

C.   Were Jack's coworkers at risk to contract AIDS from him?

NOTE: See note above about the unlikely possibility of AIDS transmission in schools. Unless Jack's coworkers had unsafe sex with him or shared needles, they would not have a risk to contract AIDS from him.

D.   How would you feel if you were a coworker of Jack's?

Case 3: A television station in the east was interviewing several people with AIDS for a news special. The station's regular camera operators refused to film these people for fear of contracting the disease. A camera team from the west coast was flown out to complete the project.

A.   Were the camera operators from the television station justified in refusing to film the people with AIDS? Why or why not?

B.   In what professions do you think people might reasonably refuse to provide services to people with AIDS?

NOTE: There are essentially no professions which should refuse services to people with AIDS. For health care personnel (doctors, dentists, nurses, etc.), standard hygiene procedures offer adequate protection against AIDS transmission.

SECTION III: REASONS FOR AND CONSEQUENCES OF PEOPLE'S DIFFERENT REACTIONS TO AIDS

A.   We have talked about some of the ways people have responded to the AIDS epidemic. It seems like there are many different responses to the same disease. Why do you suppose people react in such different ways to AIDS?

Possible answers:

1. Fears (of gay people, of disease, of death, of differences between people, etc.)

2. Level of knowledge and education (how much someone knows about AIDS and how it is transmitted, etc.)

3. Moral beliefs:

    a. If you believe it is good to help others, you might help out AIDS prevention organizations or people with AIDS.

    b. If you believe homosexuality, drug use, or sex in general is bad, you might feel you should not help out people with AIDS, or that you do not want to be involved.

4. Different personality types: optimists, pessimists, helpers, problem- solvers, complainers.

5. Past experiences: Knowing someone with AIDS or someone at risk for AIDS makes it more likely you will (1) sympathize with others with AIDS: (2) change high-risk behaviors of your own; (3) volunteer or help in some other way.

6. Others?

B. What sorts of problems might arise when people's negative judgments about homo-sexuality or IV drug users affect their reaction to AIDS?

Possible answers:

1. Not supporting research. Anyone can get AIDS under certain circumstances. Finding cures, treatments and vaccines is important for everyone.

2. Not supporting prevention or education. AIDS has created a tremendous demand on national resources—for medical research, for medical treatment, for mental health and social support services, on young and productive members of the workforce, etc. Prevention—educating people about the disease and how to stop its transmission—is the most cost-effective way to respond to the epidemic. It is the *only* way at present to stop the spread of the disease.

3. Mistreatment of and discrimination against people with AIDS, or those thought to be at risk for AIDS.

C.   DISCUSS: People reacting to AIDS through fear, misunderstanding, poor judgments, etc., creates confusion, interferes with education, slows research and hurts others. What can be done to help people understand AIDS better and react in a positive, helpful manner?

Plan 3: Civil Rights Issues Involving AIDS

Target:
Civics, social studies, history, ethics.
Classes interested in civic concerns, and/or challenged by issues without clear-cut answers.

Purpose:
1   To examine the relationship between civil liberties and public welfare, using AIDS as a current and relevant example.

2.   To communicate risk information for AIDS, risk reduction guidelines, and clarify that the AIDS virus is not spread by casual contact.

Objectives:
1.   Students will have an appreciation of the difficulties involved in guaranteeing individual freedoms while protecting public welfare.

2.   Students will know basic information about AIDS transmission.

3.   Students will know general risk-reduction guidelines for AIDS.

Format:
1.   Lecture/discussion.
2.   Written exercises (optional).
3.   Objective exam (optional).

Materials:
1.   Worksheets 1, 2, 3 or 4 (optional).
2.   Test (optional).

Time:
1-3 full class periods (at teacher's discretion).

Utilization:
Present a short lecture on AIDS. Select case examples from those given and share with students. Facilitate discussion using the suggested questions as guidelines.

Plan 3: Civil Rights Issues Involving AIDS

Method: Present the "Basic Information About AIDS" lecture. Then select one or more of the following sections for discussion.

BASIC INFORMATION ABOUT AIDS

Present the sample lecture, page 25, or your own lecture, including the following:

> What is AIDS?
> Who gets AIDS?
> How do people get AIDS?
> What is it like to have AIDS?
> What is ARC?
> How long is the incubation period for AIDS?
> What are the basic guidelines for AIDS prevention?
>   (List of safe and unsafe sexual practices—p. 23).

NOTE: For this unit, it is especially important to make clear the fact that AIDS is *not* casually transmitted, since this has significant bearing on some of the discussion issues.

SECTION I: SCHOOL AND AIDS

Daniel is a popular high school junior who has been diagnosed with AIDS. He became ill in October and was absent from school for several weeks. When he returned to school, he was fatigued but ready to continue his classes. Because he is well-known on campus, his absence was noticed by other students. He has told people that he has AIDS.

A.   Do you think Daniel should be allowed to continue to attend school? How would you feel if he was in some of your classes?

B.   Should any special provisions be made for Daniel? What do you think about his using the same cafeteria, gym, pool, locker room and bathrooms as other students?

C.   How do you think other students in our school would react if a student here were diagnosed with AIDS?

D.   Let's change the story a bit. Imagine that Daniel became sick in the summer, so people were not aware of his illness. He returned to school in the fall, looking perfectly healthy. He did not tell anyone he had AIDS. Do you think this would be okay?

E.   Would any of your feelings about this change if we were talking about a fourth grader instead of a high school student? A first grader?

F.   Some parents have insisted that they have a right to know if their children are attending school with another child who has AIDS. Do you agree?

NOTE: Informing parents would violate the privacy of the child with AIDS and his/her family, and would be illegal.

G.   Imagine that the character in our story is *Mr.* Daniels, a teacher in your school. Should he be allowed to teach? How would you feel if he were one of your teachers?

H.   What about other school personnel? If they have AIDS, should they be able to continue their work? (Consider administrators, counselors, secretaries, janitors, cafeteria workers, etc.)

I.   What kind of education about AIDS do you think is necessary in this school? What do the students here need to know about the disease? How should that information be shared with them?

SECTION II: EMPLOYER/EMPLOYEE RELATIONS AND AIDS

Sharon is a sales clerk in a clothing store. She is not actually diagnosed with AIDS. She has, however, developed medical conditions related to AIDS, called AIDS-related complex, or ARC. She feels well enough to continue working, but mentions her condition to her boss, Helen, because she will need some extra time off for medical appointments.

A.   Her boss is concerned that other people working with Sharon will be exposed to AIDS. What would you tell Helen about this?

B.   Helen has had a difficult time keeping employees for very long. She believes that when her other employees find out about Sharon's illness, they will be afraid and quit their jobs. What should Helen do?

C.   Helen overhears someone on the street saying they will not shop at the store any longer because one of the clerks there is sick with AIDS. She believes Sharon's presence in the store is hurting business. What should she do?

D.   Would you go to a store that employed someone with AIDS? A restaurant?

E.   Do you think there are any jobs that people with AIDS should not be allowed to do?

F.   Do you think there should be rules or laws protecting individual employees who may have AIDS from being fired?

G.   Do you think the business community in general has any responsibility to educate people about AIDS?

H.   What do you think the businesses in this community should do about AIDS?

SECTION III: ACCESS TO SERVICES FOR PEOPLE WITH AIDS OR ARC

Justin is a gay man with AIDS. He has Kaposi's sarcoma, and some of the lesions from the disease show on his face. He has just boarded a bus and paid his fare. The bus driver, seeing the lesions, says, "I'm not going to have you on this bus because you have AIDS. I have other passengers to protect. You will have to get off the bus." Justin refuses to get off the bus; he sits in one of the available seats. The bus driver refuses to start the bus again until Justin gets off. The other passengers begin to get angry because they are trying to get somewhere, and the bus is just sitting there. Some of them yell at the bus driver, and some of them yell at Justin.

A.   If you were one of the passengers on the bus, what would you do?

B.   What would have been the best thing for Justin to do in this situation?

C.   What would have been the best thing for the bus driver to do in this situation?

D.   Should people with AIDS be free to ride public buses?

E.   If you were manager of the bus system, what kind of policy do you think you might set for situations like this?

F.   Are there any public services you can think of (stores, restaurants, gyms, theaters, schools, health clinics, bars, national parks, etc.) that should be limited in some way for people with AIDS?

SECTION IV: FAMILIES AND AIDS

Roberto is a one-year-old boy who was adopted into a family with a mother, a father, a four-year-old brother Juan, and a six-year-old sister Maria. The family loves Roberto very much and is happy he has come to live with them. He has had a lot of health problems, which doctors could not explain for some time. Now the parents have found out that Roberto has AIDS, apparently transmitted from his biological mother, who is a user of IV drugs. Roberto has been in the hospital but is scheduled to be released soon.

A.   If you were the parents in this family, what would you do?

B.   Should Roberto be allowed to return to his home?

NOTE: There has never been a case of AIDS being transmitted within a family except (1) where there has been a sexual relationship, such as between husband and wife; and (2) in one instance where a mother of a very sick child was changing waste bags and handling a lot of feces and urine without the usual precautions (gloves, washing, etc.). It turned out the child had AIDS, and the mother has since developed antibodies to the virus. Standard hygiene precautions in such instances would prevent transmission of the virus. Many families with children have been studied, and in no instance has one child with AIDS infected any other child in the family.

C.   Do you think a parent with AIDS should be allowed to care for his or her children?

D.   A social worker involved with Roberto's case has just discovered that the boy's biological mother is pregnant again. What should be done in this instance?

NOTE: There are laws in the United States against forced sterilization or abortion. A child born to a mother infected with AIDS has about a 60% chance of also being infected. A child with AIDS can expect a limited life- span filled with much illness and multiple hospitalizations. The cost of care for such children is very high, and often is paid by public funds. This is because the mothers, if they are IV drug users, do not usually have the resources to pay for such care themselves.

SECTION V: PERSONS WHO CONSCIOUSLY TRANSMIT AIDS

A man with AIDS-related complex (ARC) was seen several times in a public clinic for treatment of gonorrhea. (Further description of ARC is found on p. 12). He admitted being sexually active with a number of different partners weekly. He was probably spreading the virus for AIDS to others in his sexual encounters.

A.   What should be done in this instance?

NOTE: Many localities have laws whereby persons who knowingly transmit diseases to others can be quarantined or detained in hospitals or correction facilities.

B.   Have you heard of other instances where someone who knew he or she had AIDS continued to expose others to the disease?

NOTE: There have been a variety of press reports of such cases.

C.   Do you think this is a common response for someone infected with the AIDS virus?

NOTE: Most people diagnosed with AIDS, and most of those who know they are at risk for the disease, are conscientious about not putting others at risk. They do not have unsafe sex, share needles, donate blood, etc. In fact, research in San Francisco shows that about 80% of gay men there have altered their sexual practices to avoid exposure to or transmission of the AIDS virus. This is a remarkable statistic, and shows a more powerful response to this health crisis than any other in history. (Consider, for example, how many people continue smoking, eat high-fat diets, refuse to wear seatbelts, etc., even though there are well-documented life-threatening risks in doing so.)

D.   Should people infected with AIDS be restricted from sexual activity? If so, what activities? If so, how should this be enforced?

NOTE: There is no reason a person infected with AIDS cannot continue to have an active and pleasurable sex life. Guidelines for safer sexual contact are clear and people following such guidelines do not pose a risk to others. For a specific list of safe and unsafe sexual activities, see page 23.

E. Occasionally, there have been suggestions of quarantining people with AIDS in some way to slow or stop the spread of the disease. Is this a useful idea? What would or would not work about this idea?

NOTE: Currently (1987), some two million people are estimated to be infected with the AIDS virus and capable of transmitting it to others. It is assumed that these people will be infectious throughout the remainder of their lives. There is no practical way to quarantine so large a number of people. Such a quarantine would be devastating to the country socially and economically. Further, there is a civil liberties issue about quarantines generally, and of restricting people's freedom when there is no evidence of any wrongdoing. The only practical answer at present is education and support for the practice of no-risk behaviors.

Plan 4: Epidemics and AIDS

Target:
> History, social studies, general science.
> Classes that enjoy discussions and are able to make deductions about different examples of similar situations.

Purpose:
> 1. To examine some historical examples of epidemics, comparing past experiences with the present-day situation of the AIDS epidemic.
>
> 2. To communicate risk information for AIDS, risk-reduction guidelines, and clarify that the AIDS virus is not spread by casual contact.

Objectives:
> 1. Students will have a sense of the historical context of epidemics and understand the AIDS epidemic in this light (in particular in terms of public reaction to past epidemics, fears of contagion, the myths that persist about epidemics).
>
> 2. Students will know basic information about AIDS transmission.
>
> 3. Students will know general risk-reduction guidelines for AIDS.

Format:
> 1. Lecture/discussion.
> 2. Written exercises (optional).
> 3. Test (optional).

Materials:
> 1. Worksheets 1, 2 or 3 (optional).
> 2. Test (optional).

Time:
> 1-3 full class periods (at teacher's discretion).

Utilization:
> Present a lecture on one or more of the epidemics described in the teaching plan, using the outline as a guide. Select appropriate items from the suggested discussion questions and facilitate the class discussion.

Plan 4: Epidemics and AIDS

Method: First, present the "Basic Information About AIDS" lecture, then present the information in Section I. Select one or more of the following sections for further lecture and discussion. Conclude the class or series of classes with discussion section 5: Looking at the AIDS Epidemic.

BASIC INFORMATION ABOUT AIDS

Present the sample lecture, page 25, or your own lecture, including the following:

> What is AIDS?
> Who gets AIDS?
> How do people get AIDS?
> What is it like to have AIDS?
> What is ARC?
> How long is the incubation period for AIDS?
> What are the basic guidelines for AIDS prevention?
>   (List of safe and unsafe sexual activities p. 23.)

SECTION I: SOME GENERAL INFORMATION ABOUT EPIDEMICS

A.   AIDS is not the only epidemic the world has ever seen, though it is one we hear a lot about right now.

B.   A medical definition of "epidemic": An illness or disease that occurs at significantly greater frequency than expected in a given population (that is, more people get it than you expect to).

C.   Some myths that have developed about epidemics:

1.   "Everyone gets sick in an epidemic."

       More people than expected get sick. There are always some people who have a natural resistance to any particular disease. There are always some people who are not exposed. Even in the worst plague epidemics of the Middle Ages, many more people lived than died.

2.   "Epidemic diseases are fatal."

       Diseases that are not necessarily fatal can still be epidemic. For example, sexually transmitted diseases (STDs or VD) are epidemic in the United States, but most are not fatal if treated medically.

61

Questions:

A.   What do you think of when you hear the word "epidemic"?

B.   What are some other myths people have about epidemics?

SECTION II: A SPECIFIC EXAMPLE: THE BUBONIC PLAGUE IN EUROPE

A.   Epidemics were common in the Middle Ages, occurring about every 25 years or so. The worst plague ever recorded in Europe was The Great Plague of 1348-1349. This was also called "The Black Death."

B.   What it was like in Europe during 1348-1349:

1.   Very high mortality: one-fourth or more of the population of Europe died (some 25,000,000 people overall).

2.   Social order collapsed: commerce stopped, food production was very low, the courts stopped meeting, there was no policing of crimes.

C.   What bubonic plague is like:

1.   Easily transmitted: people contracted bubonic plague from the bites of fleas who had gotten the infection from infected rats. Living conditions in cities were crowded and unsanitary; rats and fleas flourished. Many people were infected and the disease spread rapidly.

2.   It is a very painful disease.

3.   Universal mortality: almost everyone who got the disease died. At the time, there was no treatment and no cure.

4.   Very fast-moving: people usually died one to three days after being infected.

D.   How people responded to the disease:

1.   They did not know how it was caused.

2.   They were afraid of catching it from those already infected, so the sick were often abandoned to die alone.

3.   Many methods were used to avoid catching the disease. Some examples:

a.   Prayer to God.

b.   Devil worship.

c. Wearing amulets or charms.

d. Chanting incantations.

e. "Abracadabra": a magic word used to ward off plague.

f. Burning incense or leaves, or burning things that filled the air with foul smells.

g. Stop bathing.

h. Stop having sex.

i. Staying inside at night.

j. Some doctors recommended washing with or drinking goat urine.

4. Blaming others: In many communities in Europe, Jews were blamed for causing or deliberately spreading the plague. They were accused of poisoning wells and planning the demise of the Christian population, even though Jews were dying of plague as much as Christians. Mass persecutions were common, and hundreds of thousands of Jews were massacred throughout Europe during these times. When the plague stopped, so did the persecutions.

Questions:

A. Does it seem like any of our current ideas about epidemics might come from the European epidemics of six centuries ago?

B. Why do you suppose Jews were blamed for causing the plague?

NOTE: Jews faced powerful discrimination during this period in Europe. Without the full legal and other civil protections accorded Christians, they were an easy population to scapegoat. Authorities and the popular press of the time often participated in or encouraged these persecutions during times of plague.

C. Do you see any parallels between this European plague and the AIDS epidemic of today?

Possible answers:

1. Fear because of uncertainty or poor information about AIDS.
2. Abandoning those who are sick because of fears of contagion (an occasional occurrence with people with AIDS in medical settings, housing, or by their families).

3. Blaming gay men for the existence of the disease, suggestions that gay men are deliberately spreading AIDS, increased persecution of the gay population.

SECTION III: ANOTHER EXAMPLE: BUBONIC PLAGUE IN SAN FRANCISCO

A. Bubonic plague appeared in San Francisco in 1900. It was first diagnosed in a Chinese man.

B. Most cases were diagnosed among Chinese.

C. The San Francisco Board of Health believed Chinatown was a source of disease because of "unwholesome odors."

D. Chinese were blamed for the disease.

E. Actions taken by city, state and federal authorities:

1. Chinatown residents were placed in quarantine.

2. The city did not provide health care to residents of Chinatown.

3. No changes were made in the poverty or overcrowded conditions in China-town.

4. Chinese and Japanese could not leave California without a federally- issued medical certificate.

5. Detention camps for San Francisco's 14,000 Chinese residents began to be prepared.

6. The State Board of Health recommended that Chinatown be razed to the ground and saturated with chloride of lime and carbolic acid. The plan was not implemented before the 1906 earthquake destroyed Chinatown.

F. San Francisco's next outbreak of plague occurred in 1907. Most of the sick were Caucasian; few were Chinese. The Board of Health implemented a citywide rat-eradication program, destroying infected rats and their fleas. The disease was stopped.

Questions:

A. Why do you suppose Chinese were blamed for the 1900 outbreak of bubonic plague in San Francisco?

Possible answers:

1. Higher incidence of the disease among Chinese.

2. The Chinese experienced many forms of discrimination at that time in San Francisco. They were an easy population to scapegoat.

B. Given that bubonic plague is spread by contagious rats and fleas, do you think the quarantine of Chinatown stopped the spread of disease?

NOTE: It did not.

C. Why do you suppose more Chinese than others got the plague in 1900?

NOTE: Overcrowding and poverty led to conditions where rats and fleas flourished in Chinatown. More infected rats means more infected fleas, which means more infected people.

D. Would detention camps have stopped the spread of plague?

NOTE: No. Detaining *people* would not have helped. Only the eradication of rats and fleas helped. In fact, further crowded conditions in a detention camp could increase the incidence of the disease.

E. Do you see any parallels between this epidemic and the AIDS epidemic today?

Some examples:

1. Unnecessary precautions were taken because of uncertainty or poor information about plague; this is sometimes true with AIDS as well (for instance, hospital workers who insist on wearing gloves and masks when working with AIDS patients, even though they will *not* be exposed to the disease without them).

2. There are cases where people with AIDS are not provided with medical treatment, as was true with the Chinatown plague cases of 1900. (San Francisco, however, has been exemplary in this current epidemic, and provides excellent care for residents diagnosed with AIDS.)

3. Blaming gay men for the existence of AIDS; increased persecution of the gay population.

SECTION IV: ANOTHER EXAMPLE: SEXUALLY TRANSMITTED DISEASES AMONG AMERICAN TEENAGERS

A.   Sexually transmitted diseases, also called STDs, or sometimes VD, are usually passed from person to person during intimate sexual contact. Currently, American teenagers (and young adults) are at risk in an epidemic of STDs.

B.   One in seven teenagers currently has an STD. (85% of reported STDs are in persons 15-30 years old.)

C.   STDs can be prevented. Some methods:

    1.   Abstaining from sex altogether.

    2.   Abstaining from sex when one partner is infected with an STD.

    3.   Limiting the number of partners decreases a person's risk.

    4.   Proper use of a condom (rubber) can prevent transmission of STDs.

D.   Laws regarding medical treatment of STDs vary from state to state. In California, anyone 13 or older can be confidentially diagnosed and treated for STDs without parental consent.

More information: The STD National Hotline, (800) 227-8922.

Questions

A.   What is it like to find out you are in a risk group for an epidemic?

B.   How do you feel about teenagers generally, knowing that so many of them have STDs?

C.   Who do you think is to blame for the epidemic of STDs among young Americans?

D.   Since STDs can be prevented (by methods outlined above), why do you suppose there continues to be an epidemic of STDs?

E.   What might be done to try to end the epidemic of STDs among teenagers?

F.   Do you see any parallels between this epidemic and the AIDS epidemic?

SECTION V: LOOKING AT THE AIDS EPIDEMIC

Questions:

A.   The United States is currently experiencing an epidemic of AIDS. Has this affected you in any way? If so, how? If not, why do you suppose it has not affected you?

B.   What do you think we can learn from history that might help us, as individuals or as a nation, in coping with the AIDS epidemic?

C.   What do you think should be done for people with AIDS in our community?

D.   What sorts of things do teenagers need to know about AIDS? How could they best get that information?

NOTE: There are other interesting epidemics in U.S. history that could also be used as examples in this teaching module. The influenza epidemic in World War I killed many people and was an easily transmitted disease; in some areas it totally changed the social and civic structures. The polio epidemic in the 1950s was a source of tremendous concern. Its cause was unknown for some time, and people often took extreme and unnecessary precautions to avoid it. As with the other epidemics discussed here, fear and misunderstanding only compounded the tragedies of the diseases.

Plan 5: STDs and AIDS

Target:
Family life education, sex education, health education, general classes.

Purpose:
1. To encourage students to conceptualize AIDS as a sexually transmitted disease.

2. To clarify issues of heterosexual transmission of AIDS.

3. To communicate risk information for AIDS, risk reduction guidelines, and clarify that AIDS is not spread by casual contact.

Objectives:
1. Students will understand AIDS in the context of other sexually transmitted diseases.

2. Students will know basic information about AIDS transmission.

3. Students will know general risk-reduction guidelines for AIDS.

Format:
1. Lecture/discussion, integrated into any already-existing teaching plan on STDs.

2. Written exercises (optional).

3. Test (optional).

Materials:
1. Worksheets 2, 3 or 5 (optional).
2. Test (optional).

Time:
This material can be presented as a single class session. It can also be abbreviated so that it represents one segment of a single class lecture covering STDs generally.

Utilization:
Present a short lecture on AIDS. Select appropriate items from the suggested questions and facilitate the class discussion.

PLAN 5: STDs and AIDS

Method: Present your basic unit on sexually transmitted diseases. Then present the "Basic Information About AIDS" lecture. Select one or more of the following sections for further discussion. You might want to review Plan 4, Section 4 (p.66), which addresses the STD epidemic among American teenagers.

BASIC INFORMATION ABOUT AIDS

Present the sample lecture, page 25, or your own lecture, including the following:

> What is AIDS?
> Who gets AIDS?
> Why do people get AIDS?
> What is it like to have AIDS?
> What is ARC?
> How long is the incubation period for AIDS?
> What are the basic guidelines for AIDS prevention?
>   (List of safe and unsafe sexual activities - p. 23.)

SECTION I: AIDS AND OTHER STDs

A.   In what ways is AIDS different from other STDs?

1.   Currently, there is no cure for AIDS.

2.   AIDS is significantly more lethal than other STDs, with few persons diagnosed living more than two years.

3.   It receives much more attention from the press.

4.   People are more afraid of AIDS than of other STDs.

5.   Many heterosexuals do not consider themselves to be at risk for AIDS.

B.   In what ways is AIDS similar to other STDs?

1.   Anyone can get it if they are exposed under the proper circumstances.

2.   There is a certain amount of social stigma attached to having AIDS, as is true with other STDs.

3.   There is a carrier state to the disease, where an infected person may look and feel healthy but can transmit the disease to others.

71

4. It can be prevented.

5. AIDS is transmitted through intimate sexual contact (or the sharing of IV needles). One does not become infected from doorknobs, towels, cups, telephones, toilets, etc.

SECTION II: HETEROSEXUAL TRANSMISSION OF AIDS

For some time after AIDS was described, it seemed unlikely that it would spread in any significant way beyond the gay male population. Now we hear warnings that heterosexual transmission is also a risk.

A. Why do you suppose AIDS first appeared among large numbers of gay men?

(Gay men as a group tend to have a significantly larger number of sexual partners than heterosexuals. Larger numbers of partners means a faster spread of an STD within any population. Some people have further suggested that AIDS has affected mostly gay men because of the more common practice of anal sex among gay men. It is true that anal sex is an excellent method of transmitting AIDS; at the same time, vaginal intercourse is *also* a means of transmission and it is important not to forget this fact. In many countries, AIDS appears predominantly among heterosexuals.)

B. How would a sexually transmitted disease found mostly among gay men begin to infect a heterosexual population?

1. The disease is also transmitted among IV drug users, many of whom are heterosexual. Their sexual partners, even if not using IV drugs, may be exposed to AIDS.

2. Heterosexual women may have sexual contact with bisexual men who are infectious for AIDS; if such women become infected, they then have the potential to infect future (heterosexual) male partners (who can infect future female partners, etc.).

C. How serious is the risk of AIDS for sexually active heterosexuals likely to be?

(Sexual transmission of AIDS from men to women and from women to men is known to occur. Relative numbers of persons diagnosed with AIDS whose only risk factor is heterosexual contact have remained small—about 4% of total cases. Because of the long incubation period of the AIDS virus, it is difficult to predict whether this trend will change in the future. However, many public health experts expect that it will. Researchers expect that in the next five years at least 7,000 cases of AIDS will be reported among heterosexual men and women without other risk factors. In two recent cases of women diagnosed with AIDS, each had had only two sexual partners in the previous six years.)

D. When the herpes epidemic came to national attention, many sexually active people made significant changes in their sexual behaviors. How do you think AIDS is likely to affect people in the future? How will this affect people you know?

SECTION III: CHANGING BEHAVIORS

A. What changes will people need to make in their behaviors to prevent the further spread of AIDS?

1. Stop using IV drugs; or if using, never share needles.

2. Abstain from sex.

3. Have sex with fewer partners. (This decreases the chances of contracting AIDS, but does not eliminate the risk.)

4. Have only safer sex; that is, do not have any kind of sex that involves an exchange of semen, blood, vaginal secretions, urine or feces. Use condoms for all types of sexual intercourse. (For a specific list of safe and unsafe sexual activities, see p. 23.)

B. What is the likelihood that people will make the necessary changes to protect themselves from AIDS?

(There is no clear answer here. A San Francisco study showed that over 80% of gay men there had made significant changes in their risk behaviors to avoid exposure to or transmission of AIDS. This is a remarkable and unprecedented response to a health threat—compare, for example, the resistance of smokers to change their risk behaviors. San Francisco has the highest per capita incidence of AIDS in the nation, and most gay men in the city have many friends and acquaintances who have been diagnosed. Whether the response of this group will be repeated among other groups who do not currently share that experience is not yet known.)

C. What would keep people from making changes to protect themselves from AIDS?

1. Not knowing about AIDS, or not having information about how to prevent AIDS.

2. Not wanting to change.

3. Not believing they are really at risk for AIDS.

4. Not being able to react to a disease that might show up five or more years after the time of infection (the consequences of unsafe behaviors are too delayed).

5. Not caring about the future.

6. Not knowing anyone with AIDS, and not being affected in any way by the disease.

7. Having friends or a sexual partner who does not support the idea of changing behaviors.

D. What sorts of things might encourage people to change risk behaviors?

1. Knowing about AIDS and how to prevent it.

2. Believing that you are personally at risk for AIDS.

3. Believing that if you do change your behaviors, it will protect you from getting AIDS.

4. Knowing someone who has AIDS.

5. Knowing others who have made changes.

6. Being involved with a sexual partner who wants to practice safer sex.

SECTION IV: EVELYN AND HAROLD

Evelyn and Harold are people in their mid-twenties who are single and sexually active. They begin dating. It seems likely, after a few dates, that they will begin to have a sexual relationship. Evelyn managed to practice safer sex with her last boyfriend, John, by suggesting they use a condom and spermicidal jelly as their birth control method. Harold, however, has had a vasectomy. Evelyn is also aware that Harold sees himself as a very masculine man, and that he does not like homosexuals. She is worried about how he will react if she brings up her wish to practice safer sex because of her concerns about AIDS.

A. What do you think Evelyn should do in this situation?

B. How might Evelyn bring up the topic of safer sex?

C. How might Harold react if she says she wants to practice safer sex?

D. Imagine that Harold and Evelyn talk about safer sex, and Harold says he is absolutely not interested in using a condom, that this is why he had a vasectomy in the first place. What do you think Evelyn should do?

E. Imagine that Evelyn has had a past relationship with a bisexual man. She suspects she may have been exposed to the AIDS virus, and part of her concern in her relationship with Harold is to protect him. Do you think she could tell Harold about this? What might happen if she did?

F.   What might make this entire situation easier for both Evelyn and Harold?

NOTE: The story of Evelyn and Harold is based on the real-life experiences of a woman in circumstances like Evelyn's. In this vignette, Evelyn promotes safer sex and Harold resists.

A participant in one of our trainings commented that, true as the story may be, Harold is a poor male role model and is stereotyped. She made this excellent suggestion: Adapt the vignette, so that Evelyn is not interested in using a condom for intercourse because she has had a tubal ligation. Have Harold be the person promoting safer sex. Divide the classroom into small groups and have half work with one version of the vignette and half with the other. In a subsequent full-class discussion, the lesson could consider the impact of sex role stereotypes on individuals' efforts to protect themselves from infection.

Plan 6: The AIDS Virus

Target:
Biology, physiology, immunology, general science, general classes. No special background is necessary.

Purpose:
1. To explain how the AIDS virus operates, including its effects on the immune system and its style of replication.

2. To outline future directions in AIDS viral research.

3. To communicate risk information for AIDS, risk-reduction guidelines, and clarify that AIDS is not spread by casual contact.

Objectives:
1. Students will have a basic understanding of the AIDS virus: how it operates, its effects on the immune system and how it replicates.

2. Students will know basic information about AIDS transmission.

3. Students will know general risk-reduction guidelines for AIDS.

Format:
1. Lecture/discussion.
2. Test (optional).

Materials:
1. Test (optional).

Time:
1-2 full class sessions (at teacher's discretion).

Utilization:
Present a short lecture on AIDS. Then present the information on the AIDS virus as outlined.

PLAN 6: THE AIDS VIRUS

Method: Present the "Basic Information About AIDS" lecture. Then follow the outline as given to present information about the AIDS virus. If lab work is part of your class curriculum, please review "Infection Control Guidelines for Classes Working with Body Fluids," p. 145.

BASIC INFORMATION ABOUT AIDS

Present the sample lecture, page 25, or your own lecture, including the following:

> What is AIDS?
> Who gets AIDS?
> How do people get AIDS?
> What is it like to have AIDS?
> What is ARC?
> How long is the incubation period for AIDS?
> What are the basic guidelines for AIDS prevention?
> > (List of safe and unsafe sexual practices - p. 23.)

SECTION I: BASIC INFORMATION ABOUT VIRUSES

A.   What is a virus?

1.   A virus is a bundle of genes surrounded by a protein coating, carrying instructions for copying itself but without the mechanism for reproduction. Strictly speaking, a virus is not actually alive because it cannot reproduce itself.

2.   Must invade a living cell to reproduce itself.

3.   Smaller than any living organism. Smaller than waves of light; can only be seen with scanning electron microscopes.

B.   What are some of the ways viruses affect our lives?

1.   Human disease:

a.   Short-term, usually nonlethal diseases (colds, flu, chicken pox).

b.   Long-term, usually nonlethal diseases (herpes).

c.   Severe illnesses that may be life-threatening (various forms of hepatitis, AIDS, polio).

d.   May be involved in development of some forms of cancer.

79

2.   Animal disease:

a.   Can invade livestock, which need to be destroyed if they have certain viral infections, thereby contributing to food shortages.

b.   Can invade pets (feline leukemia, rabies and equine encephalitis all kill the animals affected).

3.   Plant diseases:

a. Destroy food crops and contribute to food shortages.

SECTION II: THREE IMPORTANT CONCEPTS ABOUT THE EFFECTS OF DISEASE-CAUSING MICRO-ORGANISMS

A.   These concepts are useful in understanding the different levels at which humans, animals or plants are affected by viruses or other micro-organisms.

1.   EXPOSURE. Actual physical contact with a disease-causing organism. Exposure does not necessarily mean an individual is infected or develops disease. If a person with a cold sneezes near you, you may be *exposed* to the virus causing the cold if any airborne moisture droplets from the sneeze reach your own mouth or nose. The cold virus may or may not enter cells in your body, causing infection or disease.

2.   INFECTION. After exposure, a disease-causing organism may invade cells in your body. This is "infection." Infection does not necessarily mean symptoms will develop. If you are exposed to and then infected with a cold virus, your immune system may be able to stop the infection before symptoms develop. Infected people, whether or not they are symptomatic, are often capable of transmitting the disease-causing organism to others.

3.   DISEASE. If, after exposure and infection, the invading organism overpowers the immune system, symptoms or disease will appear. Depending on the characteristics of the organism and your own immune system, the disease may be mild or severe.

SECTION III: THE SPECIAL CHARACTERISTICS OF THE AIDS VIRUS

A.   The AIDS virus most typically attaches itself to a type of cell called a *helper T-cell* (also called a T4 cell). Helper T-cells are a part of the immune system's first line of defense against disease, and most researchers believe the AIDS virus infects and destroys them. These cells are called "T- cells" because they are produced by the thymus gland.

On occasion, the AIDS virus will attach to other kinds of cells as well, including B-cells and macrophages, which are from different parts of the immune system.

B.   The role of helper T-cells and suppressor T-cells in the functioning of the healthy immune system.

Simply explained, the helper T-cell is a "sentry" of the immune system that moves through the body looking for foreign organisms. If a helper T-cell bumps into a foreign cell or organism, it sends alarm signals to the spleen and lymph nodes. These organs, in turn, signal other helper T-cells in the body to reproduce quickly to fight the invader. The spleen and lymph nodes also produce other specialized cells that assist in the immune response. Antibodies are produced by the B-cells.

Once the infection is under control, another kind of cell, called a *suppressor T-cell,* calls off the attack. The "alarm" is turned off and the system returns to normal.

Our bodies have gone through this process thousands of times in our lives. Usually we are never aware of the invasion because the process works well so we do not become ill.

C.   How the AIDS virus replicates.

When an AIDS virus enters the blood stream, it searches for a helper T-cell. The helper T-cell has a specific *receptor site* for the protein coating on the virus. The virus fits into the cell much like a puzzle piece. It will not fit cells that do not have this special receptor site.

The exact mechanisms of replication by the AIDS virus are not perfectly understood, but one plausible theory holds that once the virus successfully invades the helper T-cell, it lies silent within the cell. The only part of the immune system that can then recognize this virus within the living cell is another matched helper T-cell. When such a cell bumps into and attaches to the infected cell, the AIDS virus disables and invades it before it can send out an alarm. There are now two viruses, in two separate cells. The AIDS virus can replicate very slowly through this cell-to-cell, "silent invasion" process.

Eventually, some other infection occurs. Many scientists believe that when the helper T-cells receive alarm signals to reproduce and fight the new infection, those cells infected with the AIDS virus do not produce more T- cells. The virus has taken over their reproductive mechanisms and uses them now to mass produce more *virus.* These new viruses are released into the blood stream. Each virus produced goes out in search of a helper T-cell of its own. In time, the cell originally invaded will be exploded by the mass of virus and die.

When the suppressor T-cell turns off the "alarm" this time, many more helper T-cells are infected with the AIDS virus, and the immune system is less effective than it was before. More and more sentries of the immune system are being silenced and destroyed before they can alert the body to invasion.

D.   The effect of an AIDS infection on the immune system.

Usually our bodies have about twice as many helper T-cells as suppressor T-cells. In AIDS, the helper T-cells are destroyed, and the ratio of helper to suppressor cells changes. It may even reverse. Then the smaller number of helper cells will recognize an infection and even start to mobilize a defense. But before there is any significant effect, the overpopulous suppressor cells call a halt to the process. The body is left without adequate defense against disease.

SECTION IV: SOME OF THE DISEASES SEEN IN AIDS

A.   The kind of immunity affected by the AIDS virus is called *cell-mediated immunity*. The immune system has many different branches that defend against different kinds of invasions. Cell-mediated immunity responds to certain kinds of infections, and those are the diseases we see in people with AIDS. These diseases are called "opportunistic infections" because they take advantage of the "opportunity" to reproduce created by a damaged immune system.

B.   People with AIDS are affected by a wide variety of bacterial, fungal, viral and protozoal infections.

C.   What some of the most common diseases are:

1.   Pneumocystis carinii pneumonia (PCP)

PCP is the most common infection found in people with AIDS. It is caused by a parasitic protozoan called *pneumocystic carinii* that is all around us. Most of us have been exposed to PCP in our lives and carry the protozoan in our bodies in a latent (inactive) state. Our helper T-cells recognize it and keep the parasite under control without our ever getting sick or being aware of its presence. For a person with AIDS, the latent PCP may be activated and the few helper T-cells available are unable to sound an effective general alarm before the suppressor T-cells stop the defensive reaction. The person develops fever, shortness of breath and difficulty breathing, and may need hospitalization. PCP can be treated, and many people with AIDS recover from the first case of PCP. But the underlying defect in the immune system remains, and some lung tissue will be permanently destroyed. In time, the person will probably develop further cases of PCP or other diseases, and with each subsequent illness he or she will be further weakened.

2. Kaposi's sarcoma (KS).

   KS is the skin cancer you may have heard about that is associated with AIDS. Originally it was seen in older (65+ years) men of Mediterranean or African descent. It appeared as flat, purplish lesions on the skin, which were occasionally disfiguring. But the disease was rarely lethal. In AIDS, KS appears primarily in young people in a very powerful form. The lesions may multiply quickly, can grow quite large, and can affect internal organs as well as the skin. People with AIDS can die of the effects of advanced KS.

3. Herpes simplex.

   Most of us have had cold sores at one time or another caused by the common herpes virus. Usually herpes appears on mucous membranes—the mouth, genitals, and possibly the eyes. These typical herpes infections are not a sign of a damaged immune system. People with AIDS, however, can be affected by the same virus in a much more powerful fashion. The sores may appear on the skin of the buttocks or thighs, throughout the mouth and throat, or internally in the lungs or gastrointestinal tract. The herpes virus may infect the brain, causing neurologic problems like confusion or paralysis.

4. Herpes varicella-zoster.

   Most of us have also been affected by another herpes virus called herpes varicella-zoster. This virus causes chicken pox in children. The infected child develops pimple-like sores over his or her body, the immune system successfully fights the disease, and two weeks later the child feels fine. Antibodies to the virus usually keep the individual from developing further infections.

   In adults, herpes varicella-zoster causes shingles, a rash of small, very painful blisters on the skin that follows nerve pathways. Shingles may appear in people with other illnesses or people under a lot of stress. In people with AIDS, this type of herpes infection is unusually severe and may disseminate over large areas of the body.

5. Other infections.

   A variety of other diseases and infections can show up in people with AIDS. These include non-Hodgkin's lymphoma (cancer), Mycobacterium avium intracellularis (bacterial), cytomegalovirus (viral), cryptococcus (fungal), candida (fungal), and others. Some illnesses in people with AIDS are so unusual they cannot be diagnosed. In all cases, the diseases are either not found in people with healthy immune systems, or are not so severe or dangerous to those who are healthy.

D.   Other effects of the AIDS virus.

In addition to its effects on the immune system, it now appears that the AIDS virus infects the brain. Some of the diseases that appear with a depressed immune system can cause neurologic damage (e.g., toxoplasmosis, disseminated herpes). In addition to this, however, even in the absence of these diseases, the virus can affect neurologic functioning. It may cause confusion, personality changes, clumsiness, difficulties with fine and gross motor coordination, etc.

Question:

Common colds and flus are *not* opportunistic infections. These illnesses are not symptoms of significant immune system repression. Knowing what you do about how the AIDS virus replicates and how it affects people, why might a severe case of flu or similar illness be dangerous to someone who had an infection with the AIDS virus?

(In response to the nonopportunistic infection, the body would produce a large number of helper T-cells. This might further stimulate growth of the AIDS virus.)

SECTION V: THE FUTURE DIRECTION OF AIDS VIRAL RESEARCH

A.   Learning more about the origins of the virus.

Scientists are trying to track the earliest known cases of AIDS. The AIDS virus may be a recent mutation of another virus, or until recently the virus may have resided in a geographically isolated group of people who had become immune to it over time.

Most researchers believe the virus originated in Africa. The theory generally accepted now is that the virus comes from the African green monkey. These animals have been found to carry a virus remarkably similar to the human AIDS virus. Most likely, through some natural chance mutation of this AIDS-like virus in monkeys, a new organism developed which was able to cross species and infect humans. In certain parts of Africa, these animals are eaten. Perhaps through ingestion of uncooked organs, or an accidental cut while preparing the carcass, a human was first infected, and the disease has spread between humans since then.

Suggestions that the disease was passed from animals to humans through scratches or bites are not well-founded. There is no evidence that biting spreads AIDS between humans, and there is no basis for considering scratching a means of transmission.

B.   Treatment efforts:

1.   Stopping or slowing the action of the virus on the immune system.

2.   Building up the immune system.

84

3. Finding medications that will keep the virus from infecting the brain.

4. Developing treatments to keep a carrier from passing the virus on to others.

5. Vaccine.

There are no successful treatments for AIDS thus far. Further knowledge about the virus will help in these developments.

C. AIDS research may help in the understanding of other diseases that involve the iimmune system.

1. Genetic immune deficiency problems (illnesses children might be born with, e.g. Wiskott-Aldrich, Severe Combined Immunodeficiency [SCID]).

2. Other acquired immune deficiency problems (organ transplants, people receiving cancer treatments, patients on steroid medications).

3. Cancer (where the immune system does not recognize a tumor or cannot effectively stop its growth).

4. Autoimmune disorders:

   a. Rheumatoid arthritis (the immune system attacks the tissues and bones around the joints, improperly identifying them as invaders).

   b. Systemic lupus erythematosus (the immune system destroys skin, kidneys, joints).

5. Allergies (the immune system responds unnecessarily to benign invaders like pollen, dust, certain foods, etc.).

Questions:

A. You can see that AIDS research is important to medical science. What are some of the things that might interfere with the progress of this research?

1. Inadequate funding.

2. Poor understanding about the benefits of the research, so that legislators and the general public do not support funding.

3. People's negative emotional reactions to AIDS (because of fear, because they blame the disease on homosexuals or IV drug users), which cause them to withhold support for such research.

4. Competition among researchers, interfering with cooperative efforts.

5. Treatment trials involve human subjects and there are many ethical problems in such research. Researchers must take into consideration the possibility of a treatment causing more damage than good, and balance this against the desperate need of people with AIDS/ARC for successful treatments.

B. Imagine that this class was actually a group of legislators about to vote on funding AIDS research. You have $1 million to disburse (remember, research is very expensive). What areas of research (as covered in Section 4, above) would you want to support? How would you convince others of your position?

Plan 7: Pursuing a Medical Mystery--
The Story of AIDs

Target:
Biology, physiology, general science.
Classes enjoying discussion and interested in scientific strategies.

Purpose:
1. To describe some of the epidemiologic tools used to identify and describe a new disease, using AIDS as a current and relevant example.

2. To communicate risk information for AIDS, risk-reduction guidelines, and clarify that the AIDS virus is not spread by casual contact.

Objectives:
1. Students will have a basic understanding of the process of epidemiology.
2. Students will know basic information about AIDS transmission.
3. Students will know general risk-reduction guidelines for AIDS.

Format:
1. Lecture/discussion.
2. Test (optional).

Materials:
1. Test (optional).

Time:
1-3 full class sessions (at teacher's discretion).

Utilization:
Present the story of the early investigations of AIDS and then facilitate discussion of how some of the early questions in the AIDS epidemic were answered by epidemiologic methods. Conclude the class with a review of AIDS risk and prevention information.

PLAN 7: PURSUING A MEDICAL MYSTERY--THE STORY OF AIDS

Method: Present the story of the early investigations of AIDS as outlined in sections I-IV. Section V offers several questions asked by researchers early in the epidemic, which were answered by epidemiologic method. Select as many of these examples as time allows for class discussion. Conclude the class with the review of AIDS risk and prevention information in Section VI.

If lab work is part of your class curriculum, please review "Infection Control Guidelines for Lab Classes Working with Body Fluids," page 145 .

INTRODUCTION:

Most students have heard about AIDS. AIDS is a relatively new disease, and a look at the history of AIDS investigations offers an exciting example of one of the ways science works.

SECTION I: THE APPEARANCE OF THE DISEASE

A.   In 1981, a perplexed physician diagnosed five presumably healthy young men in Los Angeles with Pneumocystis carinii pneumonia (PCP).

   1.   PCP is a disease caused by a parasitic protozoan. It is a very serious disease seen only in people with depressed immune systems.

   2.   Having a depressed immune system (being "immunocompromised" or "immune suppressed") indicates severe damage to the immune system.

B.   Coincidentally, all five men were homosexuals.

C.   The doctor reported these unusual cases to the Centers for Disease Control in Atlanta (CDC).

   1.   The CDC is a national center, under the direction of the U.S. Public Health Service, that studies the distribution and incidence of disease in the United States and researches causes and cures.

   2.   The CDC has the ability to require that certain diseases be reported to them when diagnosed.

D.   The CDC published the report of the Los Angeles doctor in the June 5, 1981 issue of Morbidity and Mortality Weekly Reports (MMWR), a widely-read publication on the occurrence of diseases in the U.S. They included the suspicion in these cases that there might be a connection between sexual contacts and the suppression of the immune system necessary for a person to be diagnosed with PCP.

E.   At the same time, 26 cases of Kaposi's sarcoma (KS) were reported among homosexual men in New York and California.

1.   KS is a skin cancer usually seen in a nonmalignant form among older men of Mediterranean or African descent.

2.   At the time of this 1981 report, eight of the 26 men diagnosed had died—a most unusual outcome with KS.

3.   The new cases of KS seemed related to immune suppression.

SECTION II: STARTING SURVEILLANCE ON AIDS

A.   *Disease surveillance* is a way of studying a disease by seeing how many cases there are, what kinds of people are getting the disease, where these people live, what kinds of things they might have in common, how they are affected by the disease, whether they live or die.

1.   Why use surveillance?

a.   To see how serious a disease is by measuring how many people get it, how seriously affected they are, whether they live or die.

b.   To try to determine causes of a disease by looking for commonalities among those affected.

c.   To understand the natural history of a disease by watching its progression in a large number of people.

B.   The CDC began systematic surveillance of individuals with KS or PCP in June, 1981.

C.   CDC looked for others who might be affected by the same disease.

1.   Since it was a new disease, they needed to tell physicians what to look for. They had to come up with a definition.

2.   Definition first used: KS or other life-threatening opportunistic infections in previously healthy people between the ages of 15 and 60.

3.   Diagnoses of the disease were required to be reported to the CDC.

SECTION III: THE DISEASE SPREADS

A.   In fall 1981, new cases of the disease were reported among male and female heterosexuals who used IV drugs.

B.   Reports were made of hemophiliacs with AIDS.

1.   Hemophilia is a disorder in which a person's blood is unable to clot after a wound. It is treated by replacing an element missing in the person's blood, called "factor VIII." Factor VIII is manufactured from donated blood.

C.   Researchers began to suspect the disease was transmitted through blood products.

D.   Several recent Haitian immigrants were also reported with the disease.

E.   Some babies were being born with hard-to-explain immunodeficiencies, and were suspected of having the disease.

F.   The incidence of the disease continued to increase.

SECTION IV: EPIDEMIOLOGY—ANSWERING QUESTIONS ABOUT AIDS

A.   The new disease was eventually called AIDS—Acquired Immune Deficiency Syndrome. (The problem with the immune system is not a genetic one, but an acquired one.)

B.   The definition was updated: The presence of KS, PCP or other opportunistic infection in a person who has no known underlying cause for immunosuppression.

C.   There was no test available to prove infection. There were many questions about transmission, cause, course of the disease, how many people would ultimately be infected, how to prevent infection, etc., which needed to be answered. Questions were raised and strategies planned to find the answers.

Today, we know that AIDS is caused by a virus and we have identified that virus. We can perform a simple test to check for the antibody to the AIDS virus. (A positive antibody test verifies infection with the virus, though it does not necessarily mean the individual will develop AIDS. Persons with positive antibody tests are presumed to be carriers, capable of passing the virus on to others in unsafe sexual exchanges or IV drug use.) For research purposes, a test for virus is also used, though this is at present very costly and difficult to perform.

The virus that causes AIDS was not discovered until 1983-1984. The antibody test was not available for use until 1985. Before this time, we relied on studies of the health and sexual practices, lifestyles, and health histories of those who had AIDS to answer many of our questions. We also looked at the distribution of the disease and compared those with AIDS to those without it.

D.   This sort of study of the distribution and causes of diseases is called "epidemiology." Surveillance is one of the tools of epidemiology.

SECTION V: DISCUSSION—QUESTIONS, STRATEGIES AND ANSWERS

Present one or more of the following questions to the class and discuss possible strategies to find the answers. Then clarify what methods were actually used in the investigations ("Strategies"), the results of the investigations ("Answers"), and how accurate those results have remained as our skills and tools for investigation improved ("Update").

Question 1: *How was AIDS being transmitted among gay men? Was it indeed sexually transmitted? Were certain sexual activities more likely to transmit the disease than others?*

Strategies: Get in-depth sexual histories from those diagnosed with the disease. Compare gay men diagnosed with AIDS with those who did not have the disease to look for differences in sexual practices. Compare the sexual practices of gay men with those of other people.

Answers: Some of the men originally diagnosed with AIDS in Los Angeles and New York were acquainted and had been past sexual partners. This strongly supported the possibility of sexual transmission.

The gay men first diagnosed with AIDS had certain sexual experiences in common, most notably anal sex with multiple partners. Gay men who did not have sex that involved an exchange of semen were not diagnosed with the disease.

An early comparison of diagnosed and nondiagnosed gay men showed that those with AIDS had higher numbers of sexual partners per year.

Update: Viral studies have now shown the presence of the AIDS virus in semen. We have further verification, through the increased numbers of gay men affected, that those who contract AIDS have a history of sexual contact involving an exchange of semen. Antibody studies have tracked a few individuals who were antibody negative (uninfected) up to a time when they engaged in unsafe sex, at which point they became antibody positive (infected). Infection via sexual activity is proven.

We now know that it is not necessary to have multiple partners to become infected with the AIDS virus. A one-time unsafe exposure may be enough to cause infection.

Question 2: *Could AIDS be passed through casual contact?*

Strategies: Look at large numbers of people who had casual contact with people with AIDS—nonsexual friends, family members, medical personnel. See if any of them came down with the disease.

Look at those diagnosed with the disease. Were there any cases of people developing AIDS whose only risk was casual contact?

Answers: Studies of friends, family members, and medical personnel showed no transmission through casual contact.

There were unanswered questions about the risks of some of those affected, but in no case were researchers able to verify casual transmission of AIDS.

Update: These studies are consistent with those ongoing today. There continue to be no documented cases of casual contact transmission. With our more sophisticated understanding of the virus now, we can be further reassured that AIDS is transmitted only through intimate sexual contact involving an exchange of blood, semen, vaginal secretions (and possibly urine and feces), or in other cases such as IV drug use where there is an exchange of blood.

Question 3: *Just how serious was this disease likely to be? In the beginning, only a few people were diagnosed as having AIDS. Would the number of cases increase slowly or dramatically?*

Strategies: Keep count of all the cases reported. See if the numbers were growing. If there was an increase in the number of cases each month (or every six months), plot a graph to make a projection of the numbers of cases expected in the future.

Answers: Ongoing counts of AIDS cases showed a definite increase in the number of cases. After the disease was identified in 1981, researchers tracked people who had shown the disease as early as 1979. Between the second half of 1979 and the first half of 1983, the number of new cases reported was doubling about every six months. Future projections of incidence were staggering—using this formula, the 1,118 cases reported in the first six months of 1983 suggested there would be over 76,000 new cases by the first six months of 1986, and over 150,000 cases overall.

Update: AIDS has indeed affected people at an alarming rate. The increase in rate of infection continues, but has slowed since the time of the earliest studies. After 1983, the number of new cases reported increased by roughly 30% every six months. In 1987, new cases are expected to double every 13 months.

We note that these figures are still quite alarming. At the time of this writing, for example, AIDS is the leading cause of death among men aged 30 to 39 in New York City, and it is the second leading cause for women there aged 30 to 34.

Question 4: *AIDS was being transmitted through infected blood donated for blood transfusions. How was the blood supply to be made safe?*

Strategies: Gay men with multiple sex partners were asked not to donate blood.

There was no test for the AIDS virus, but the blood of those diagnosed with AIDS could be examined for other elements for which a test might exist. If there were such elements, blood could be screened by whatever test already existed.

Answers: Studies showed that most people with AIDS also had antibodies to hepatitis-B, a disease also passed through blood exchange and intimate sexual contact. An antibody test existed for hepatitis-B, and its use was instituted at blood banks. Combined with voluntary screening by gay men, 90% of AIDS- infected blood was successfully removed from the blood supply.

Update: The development of the AIDS antibody test in 1985 has further improved the safety of the blood supply. Almost all infected blood is now able to be screened out. The chance of an infected unit of blood passing through the screening process is estimated to be about 1 in 100,000. (Actually, the National Academy of Sciences gives a range of estimates, presenting the most pessimistic risk as 1 in 20,000, the most optimistic as 1 in 1,333,000, and the baseline as 1 in 99,000.) Though the risk of AIDS via transfusion still remains, it is a much smaller risk than the risk of not accepting a transfusion in cases in which it is medically necessary to do so.

Question 5: *How long is the incubation period for the disease? It seemed it might be several months at the outset of investigations. This was considered quite lengthy.*

Strategies: It was difficult to measure incubation for a sexually transmitted disease with a long incubation rate. Often people had had several sexual partners and many possible exposures in any six-month period of time.

People who developed AIDS after transfusions were easier to measure for incubation, because usually there was only one time when blood was transfused, and that time was recorded in medical records.

Answers: Tracking transfusion-related AIDS cases gave definite answers, but the disease kept showing longer and longer periods of incubation. Incubations of four or more years were proven in this method.

Update: With the advent of the antibody test, stored blood serum samples could be tested for infection with the AIDS virus. Several thousand gay men donated blood samples in 1978 and 1979 for use in the development of a vaccine for hepatitis-B. Hundreds of those men are under study today, and subsequent blood samples have been collected and studied for AIDS infection. We now know that some men who showed AIDS infection in their 1978 samples of blood have developed the disease as much as seven years later. The average incubation is estimated, in 1987, to be over five years.

Question 6: *Why were newborns developing AIDS?*

Strategies: Look for risk factors for the newborns. Had they received blood transfusions?

Was it possible that the mothers were infected and had passed the disease to their babies before or shortly after birth?

Answers: Babies diagnosed with AIDS did show risk factors. Many had received transfusions in the newborn period. Others were children of mothers who used IV drugs. A few were children of Haitian women, though the risk for Haitians was not well understood at the time (see #7, below). It seemed probable that the children were infected with AIDS before birth, incubating the disease for a short period of time and then becoming ill, usually in the first year of life.

Update: This is further verified by viral and antibody studies. Newborns of mothers known to carry the AIDS virus have been tested at birth, and about half have the AIDS virus. Of those infants who *are* infected, most have developed illness within six months of birth.

Question 7: *Why were Haitians being infected with AIDS?*

Strategies: Most Haitians with AIDS denied homosexuality or IV drug use. It was necessary to look for other possible courses of transmission as well as consider the possibility that the reporting by those diagnosed was inaccurate. Most of the initial questioning was done by Caucasian researchers unfamiliar with Haitian culture. Perhaps a Haitian researcher could get different answers.

Answers: When those familiar with Haitian culture were brought into the investigation, several important points came to light. One was that there was a strong cultural judgment against homosexuality, so that many gay Haitians denied their sexual orientation. Another was the fact that in Haiti, a very poor country, some men who considered themselves heterosexual would act as male prostitutes for gay tourists in the cities. Because this was work performed to earn money, the men did not consider it "homosexual activity." Further, a man who was the active rather than receptive partner in anal sex would not, in Haiti, consider himself a homosexual. Finally, many Haitians used the services of folk healers who administered injections of folk remedies with needles that were not properly sterilized, hence there was evidently blood transmission of AIDS.

This collection of information seemed to answer many of the questions about Haitian risk.

Update: Now that we understand the possibilities of heterosexual transmission, it is evident as well that many of the AIDS infections among Haitians were passed through heterosexual contact.

Question 8: *Gay men diagnosed with AIDS sometimes had sexual partners who seemed perfectly healthy. Was there a carrier state for the disease, in which people appeared healthy but could pass the disease to others?*

Strategies: Monitor the partners of people with AIDS to determine whether they eventually developed the disease. Look at the previous and subsequent partners of these men to see if they developed AIDS.

Answers: This was a difficult study to pursue because of the length of incubation and the difficulty of determining who a carrier might be in a population in which many people have multiple sexual partners. It was true that sexual partners of people with AIDS often developed the disease at a later date. Generally, the studies seemed to suggest there was a healthy carrier state, or a period during the incubation of the disease in which a person appeared normal but could infect others.

Update: Again, antibody and viral studies have clarified this question. There is no longer any doubt about the carrier state for AIDS. Many people look quite healthy and can still pass the virus.

Question 9: *Were the heterosexual partners of IV drug users at risk, even if they did not themselves use IV drugs?*

Strategies: Monitor the sexual partners of IV drug users diagnosed with AIDS to see if they develop the disease.

Answers: AIDS evidently could be passed heterosexually between IV drug users and their nonusing partners. Some men and women with no other risk than sexual contact with an IV user developed AIDS.

Update: This is further verified by antibody studies of IV drug users and their sexual partners. Depending on the study, anywhere from 10% to 70% of nonusing partners may be infected.

Question 10: *Were heterosexuals generally at risk to contract the disease, if they did not have a history of IV drug use or homosexuality?*

Strategies: Look at all the people diagnosed with AIDS and see if heterosexual contact was the only possible risk for any of them.

Answers: The disease spread most rapidly among IV drug users and gay men, but it appeared in some places among heterosexuals without other known risk factors. There were cases of AIDS passing from men to women, as well as those showing transmission from women to men. Heterosexuals were also susceptible to the disease.

Update: This trend continues. In the U.S., sexually active heterosexuals with no other risk factor account for a small but growing number of AIDS cases.

SECTION VI: THE FUTURE DIRECTION OF AIDS EPIDEMIOLOGY

A.   In the future, more sophisticated tools will be available for studying AIDS. For example, it is possible that soon there will be a good, inexpensive test to determine presence of virus (current viral tests are costly and difficult, and are only used for research). This will allow for more effective screening of blood supplies and more accurate research. (There are some limitations with the currently available antibody test.)

B.   Epidemiological studies will continue and will look especially at the following:

    1.   To determine the origins of the virus. If we know where the virus originated and can see it in earlier forms, we may find clues to treatment or the development of a vaccine.

    2.   To monitor changes in people being affected by AIDS. Increased educational outreach to IV drug users and sexually active heterosexuals is being implemented because changes in the pattern of infection suggest growing risk in these groups.

    3.   To study whether treatments work: comparing those receiving a treatment with those receiving a placebo.

    4.   To test a vaccine if one is successfully developed, especially to see if it is effective and safe before it is widely used.

    5.   To monitor the different ways the disease affects different people (for example, fewer people are now being diagnosed with KS than was originally the case; and KS rarely affects anyone with AIDS who is not also a gay man).

    6.   To monitor people who have survived with an AIDS diagnosis for several years, trying to discover how they have managed to battle this usually fatal disease.

SECTION VII: REVIEW

A.   Since so much effort has gone into understanding AIDS, we review here the information discovered that might be important in the lives of students.

    1.   *Anyone* can get AIDS. It is not a gay disease. It can pass from men to men, from men to women, and from women to men.

    2.   You can't tell just by looking at someone whether he or she has been infected with AIDS.

    3.   You can prevent exposure to AIDS by following simple guidelines:

a. Don't use IV drugs. If you must use drugs, don't *ever* share needles with anyone! (We also recommend that you do not share needles for tattooing or piercing ears because of the possible risk of blood exchange.)

b. Don't engage in sexual activity. Be abstinent.

c. If you do choose to be sexually active, follow safer sex guidelines at all times. This means don't exchange blood, semen, vaginal secretions, urine or feces in any sexual activity. Condoms, properly used, prevent exposure to the AIDS virus. (For a specific list of safe and unsafe sexual activities, see p. 23.)

4. Testing of donated blood has made the blood supply quite safe, so transfusion-related AIDS will be very rare in the future.

5. Blood products for people with hemophilia are now heat-treated to kill the AIDS virus, so hemophiliacs are no longer exposed to AIDS in medical treatment.

Supplement:
How the AIDS Virus
Infects the Immune System

This supplement is provided to assist teachers in explaining the process of infection by the AIDS virus to classes interested in this information. It describes in a graphic and simple manner the effects of AIDS on the immune system.

(Diagrams 2-A and 2-B (p. 100) are available as teaching aids for this supplement.)

A.   The immune system is a very complicated system through which the body defends itself from invasion by diseases and infection. AIDS acts by destroying the body's immune system and opening the body up to certain infections that would normally be stopped by the immune system.

Two of the infections which are seen in people with AIDS are Pneumocystis carinii pneumonia (PCP) and Kaposi's sarcoma (KS). People with healthy immune systems *never* get these diseases. (Other conditions besides AIDS can damage the immune system; in such cases, these diseases might also appear.)

B.   **The Healthy Immune System** (Diagram 2-A):

The different parts of the immune system work together to protect the body. The body can fight certain diseases *all* the time. It can fight other diseases *most* of the time.

In this diagram, you can see the healthy immune system successfully fighting PCP and KS. Some cases of flu are stopped, but occasionally a flu or cold might take hold.

The part of the immune system shown by dots in the diagram is the *helper T- cells*. They act as sentries, alerting the body to invasion by diseases like PCP and KS.

C.   **The Immune System Infected with AIDS** (Diagram 2-B):

The AIDS virus destroys helper T-cells. You can see that the person with AIDS has very few helper T-cells. The body can no longer fight off diseases like PCP or KS. It may be able to fight off infections like flu or cold.

D.   Another way to think about this:

Think of the body as a castle, with defending armies inside (the immune system) and attacking armies outside (diseases). A spy (AIDS virus) comes into the castle and destroys all the sentries (the helper T-cells) of the defending armies. When diseases attack, no sentries are left to warn the defending armies. The troops are not alerted to the invasion, and the immune system is easily overwhelmed by the attackers.

2-A: THE HEALTHY IMMUNE SYSTEM

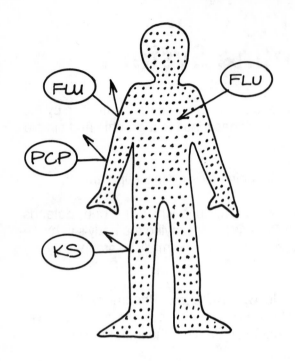

The body's immune system can <u>always</u> fight off certain diseases, including PCP and KS. It can usually, but not always, fight common colds or flu.

:::: -   Helper T-cells: special cells in the immune system which alert the body to invasion by diseases.

FLU -   Common viral colds or flus.

PCP-   Pneumocystis carinii pneumonia: a disease seen in some people with AIDS.

KS -   Kaposi's sarcoma: also seen in some people with AIDS.

2-B: THE IMMUNE SYSTEM INFECTED WITH AIDS

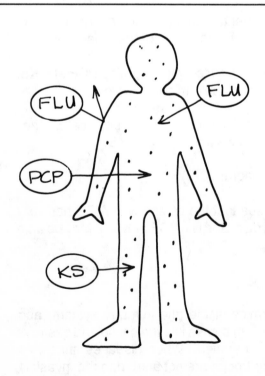

The AIDS virus has destroyed most of the helper T-cells.

The body cannot fight off diseases like PCP and KS. It can sometimes, but not always, fight common colds and flu.

TEACHING MATERIALS

Introduction to Teaching Materials

The materials provided in this curriculum are optional additions to the class lectures and discussions. They can be assigned as homework or filled out in a subsequent class session. There are six worksheets and an objective test included.

1.   **Personal Opinions About AIDS**

This is a preclass worksheet. Students are asked to spend a few minutes filling out the worksheet at the beginning of class. Since the worksheet asks for opinions, there are no right or wrong answers. Students should not put their names on the worksheet. At the end of the class, the students are asked to look over their answers and, if they feel differently about any of them, change them. Then they are instructed to turn over the sheet and write on the back the most important thing they learned in the class.

2.   **People's Responses to AIDS**

This worksheet allows students to consider which responses to the AIDS epidemic they consider positive, and which they consider negative. It is a simple exercise, appropriate for all high school levels.

3.   **Press Reports on People's Responses to AIDS**

Worksheet 3 involves an evaluation of responses to AIDS reported in the press. It requires the student to find an article about AIDS in a newspaper or magazine. As an alternative the teacher could give students a copy of a particularly useful article and have them answer the questions about that article specifically. This is also a fairly simple exercise, appropriate for all high school levels.

4.   **Finding Answers to Questions About AIDS**

This worksheet absolves the teacher from the responsibility of knowing everything there is to know about AIDS! Any unanswered questions students have can be pursued with the help of this worksheet. This also allows students to pursue questions they might be hesitant to raise in class. The teacher should check for the name and phone number of a local AIDS information switchboard, or use the national information number listed on page 153 , and enter this on the worksheet before making copies for students. Resource numbers *do* change sometimes, so be sure to check the number before handing out the exercise.

We recommend that this worksheet be handed out in all classes, even as an optional exercise, so students can take the information number home and use it privately if they wish.

5. **Setting Policy About AIDS**

Worksheet 5 involves essay answers to some complex and challenging questions about AIDS policies. It is a more difficult worksheet than the previous three, will take more time to complete, and is appropriate for students accustomed to critical and analytic thinking and writing.

6. **An AIDS Education Plan**

The task of worksheet 6 is also challenging. If preferred, it could be done as a class or small group project rather than individually. The results of the work might actually be shared with school administrators, school board, etc., as a way of involving students in the issue.

Test

The 10-question objective test covers AIDS transmission and prevention, as well as some basic information about the disease. It is appropriate in any class needing measurement of class comprehension for evaluation of students or teachers, or for grading purposes. The test can also be given as a pretest, then given again after the unit, as a way to show students what they have learned.

Worksheet 1
Personal Opinions About AIDS

These are personal opinion questions. There are no wrong answers! Please answer as honestly as you can. Do not put your name on this paper.

1.   I think people with AIDS ————————————————————

_____

_____

_____

2.   Learning about AIDS in school is:

    a.   A good idea. Really important.

    b.   A bad idea. A waste of time.

    c.   Other ————————————————————

_____

3.   Is there any way the AIDS epidemic has affected you, or might affect you in the future?

_____

_____

_____

_____

Worksheet 2
People's Responses to AIDS

1.   Think of someone you know or someone you have heard of who has responded to the AIDS epidemic in a way you feel is positive and helpful.

What has his or her response to the AIDS epidemic been?

_____

_____

Why do you think this is a positive and helpful response?

_____

_____

_____

2.   Think of someone you know or someone you have heard of who has responded to the AIDS epidemic in a way you feel is negative and not helpful.

What has his or her response to the AIDS epidemic been?

_____

_____

Why do you think this response is negative and not helpful?

_____

_____

_____

Worksheet 3
Press Reports on People's Responses to AIDS

Find an article about AIDS in a newspaper or magazine that talks, at least in part, about people and AIDS. (Articles reporting only research news may not mention anything about people, and would not be useful for this exercise.) Attach the article to this worksheet and answer the following questions:

1.　Who are the people (or the person, or the groups) mentioned in this article?

_____

_____

_____

2.　How are these people (or this person, or these groups) responding to the AIDS epidemic?

_____

_____

_____

3.　How do you feel about what these people (this person) are doing? Do you think their responses are positive? Negative? Do you agree or disagree with what they are doing? Why?

_____

_____

_____

_____

Worksheet 4
Finding Answers to Questions About AIDS

1. Think of a question you have about AIDS that has not been answered in the class. Write the question:

   _____

   _____

   _____

2. The AIDS information number is _____. Call this number and ask your question. Write the answer to the question:

   _____

   _____

   _____

3. What was the person who answered your call like? Helpful? Clear? Hard to understand?

   _____

   _____

4. Would you call the switchboard again if you had another question about AIDS?
   ____ Yes ____ No
   Why or why not?

   _____

   _____

   _____

Worksheet 5
Setting Policy About AIDS

Four fictional situations in which someone must respond in some way to an AIDS-related issue are given below. Choose one of these situations and write a response, keeping in mind the need to protect the civil rights of all parties involved.

1. You are the principal of an elementary school of 300 students. It is July, and you have just been informed that one of the sixth graders returning to school in September has been diagnosed with AIDS. What will you do?

2. You are the Director of Parks and Recreation for a large city. A group of people with AIDS has requested use of [...] event. This permission is often granted [...] however, a newspaper prints a report of [...] erupts. Many citizens claim this org [...] pool and endanger the health of othe [...]

3. You are the Director of Adm [...] you have an application from a man whic [...] accepted into the school, although his [...] One of your employees says he has pe [...] You know if this is true, the man is not li [...] Placements in your school are few, and [...]

4. You are a counselor at a so [...] meet with you. She has a history of IV drug [...] he has been ill, and as she describes h [...] have AIDS-related complex (ARC). She tells you she is trying [...] that she and her husband are very excited about starting a family together. What will you do?

[handwritten note overlaying text: "Please type this DONE on separate sheet and give to Pete, replies,"]

113

Worksheet 6
An AIDS Education Plan

Imagine that the principal of this school has hired you to make sure that all the students in this school know about AIDS—what it is, how it is transmitted, and how it can be prevented. Write a proposal explaining to the principal how you think this can best be done.

_____

_____

_____

_____

_____

_____

_____

_____

_____

_____

_____

_____

_____

_____

Test

Circle the best answer for each question.

1. Who can get AIDS?

   a. Gay men.
   b. People with hemophilia.
   c. Anyone.

2. Which of these activities never spreads AIDS?

   a. Having intercourse without a condom.
   b. Donating blood.
   c. Sharing IV needles in drug use.

3. You cannot tell by looking at someone whether he or she has AIDS.

   a. True
   b. False

4. What is one important way to reduce your risk for AIDS?

   a. Make sure your sexual partner looks healthy.
   b. Don't hug IV drug users.
   c. Use safer sex.

5. What is safer sex?

   a. Look for spots on your partner's body.
   b. Don't exchange blood, semen or vaginal secretions.
   c. Only have sex once in a while.

6. Which of these is a way the AIDS virus is transmitted?

   a. On toilet seats.
   b. Someone coughing.
   c. Intimate sexual contact.

7. A woman who once used IV drugs stopped doing so about two years ago. She feels perfectly healthy. Does she need to worry about the possibility of her sexual partner getting AIDS from her?

   a. Yes.
   b. No.

8. Condoms, when properly used, can protect you from infection with the AIDS virus.

   a. True.
   b. False.

9. Which of these activities might expose you to AIDS?

   a. Eating at a restaurant that employs a gay cook.
   b. Getting an amateur tattoo from a friend.
   c. Using a public drinking fountain.

10. Which of the following is in a high risk group for AIDS?

    a. Asian women.
    b. Babies born to parents who use IV drugs.
    c. Women who take tranquilizers.

Answer key:

    1. c
    2. b
    3. a
    4. c
    5. b
    6. c
    7. a
    8. a
    9. b
    10. b

BACKGROUND MATERIALS

Lingering Doubts About Casual Transmission

We believe that students are best served by clear and unambiguous information about AIDS. It is most useful, therefore, if we can agree about the major facts on AIDS, and teachers can present the material with confidence. However, a concern we hear fairly often is the possibility that AIDS might be transmitted by casual contact. In all our materials, we insist that it is not, but if a teacher disagrees with this, how is he or she to teach the curriculum?

We offer here some of the arguments for and against casual transmission. We hope this will clarify the issue further.

"There is so much we don't know about AIDS. How can we be sure of anything?"

Actually, we know a great deal about AIDS. We know it is caused by a virus, and we know quite a bit about the structure of this virus. We understand how the virus attacks the immune system, and we have seen that it is fragile and dies easily outside the human body. We are familiar now with the progression of the disease and the range of illnesses that appear in infected persons. From a variety of studies, we understand that AIDS is transmitted only in circumstances where blood is exchanged, or where there is intimate sexual contact involving an exchange of blood, semen, vaginal secretions (and possibly urine or feces). What we do not know is how to stop the progress of the disease, how to cure it, or how to vaccinate against it.

"The incubation period for AIDS is so long. How can you be sure a lot of people who have had casual contact with persons with AIDS are not in that period of incubation? The disease could appear years from now."

The incubation period for AIDS, often five years or more, is long. However, the length of time between an infection and the development of antibodies is fairly short, usually taking only two to twelve weeks.

Many antibody studies have been performed on family members of people with AIDS who share "casual contact," and there has never been a spread of infection. Perhaps even more persuasive are the studies of health care workers who care for people with AIDS every day. Many medical personnel have been working with people with AIDS for several years. They are often in very close contact with those infected, giving them shots, performing exams, bathing them, cleaning linen and disposing of body wastes. Simple and standard precautions are followed, like washing hands after physical examination, wearing gloves while disposing of body wastes, etc.

121

An article in a July, 1987, medical journal (Journal of Infectious Diseases) summarized reports on over 2,400 health and dental care workers who had been tested for AIDS antibodies. Of these, 817 had had parenteral (within blood veins) or mucous membrane exposure to blood or other body fluids from people with HIV infection. Occupational exposure was clearly documented in one case in which a worker was actually injected with blood which had been drawn from a person with AIDS, and three other cases of possible occupational exposure through accidental needlesticks were reported. In addition, there are now a few other reports of caregivers becoming infected: one worker with chapped hands placed direct pressure on an open wound for about 20 minutes, having prolonged exposure to the patient's blood; another had copious splashes of blood in the eyes and on open sores on the skin; in one case a mother caring for a sick child had regular direct contact with the child's bloody feces and other body excretions.

The development of HIV infection in these people is disturbing, though the greater surprise is that with this many documented accidental exposures (over 800), we do not see more cases of infection. Every one of these cases could have been avoided had infection control guidelines been followed consistently. These studies further verify that AIDS is not transmitted in casual, day-to-day contact, but it may be transmitted in unusual circumstances where there is very direct or prolonged exposure to infected blood or waste products.

We hope all health care providers will follow infection control guidelines in any patient contact in the future. (The guidelines are outlined on p. 143.)

"About 3% of AIDS cases in the United States have 'no known risk factor.' Where did these several hundred people get AIDS, if not through the usual risk activities reported?"

Reporting on a disease diagnosed in 40,000+ modern-day Americans is a true challenge. Those affected are dispersed over the entire country, and they are treated in a variety of medical settings. Accurate reporting in these circumstances is always difficult. Remember that 97% of AIDS cases have a known risk factor consistent with the information we have presented in this curriculum. The other 3% are entered into a category called "none of the above/other," which is not actually the same as "no known risk." Here is where most of those 3% fall:

1. Early on in the AIDS epidemic, Haitian immigrants were listed as a risk category. Since that time, this category has been removed from the official reports on AIDS published by the Centers for Disease Control. Almost half of the 3% of cases in the "Other" category are Haitians diagnosed with AIDS. There are three likely modes of transmission among this population: (1) heterosexual contact; (2) sharing of IV needles in the administration of medicines by folk healers; and (3) male homosexual contact unreported because of different cultural understandings about what constitutes homosexuality, or because of antihomosexual feelings in the culture.

2. Some people are diagnosed with AIDS and fail to return for follow-up questioning

to determine risk factors. This is not uncommon among transient or highly mobile groups, which many IV drug users and some gay men are. These people are entered into the "other" category.

3.   Some individuals are diagnosed with AIDS after death. Risk information is often unavailable in these cases.

4.   Some people diagnosed with AIDS are too ill at the time of diagnosis to provide information about themselves. Others do not want to provide the information.

5.   The major risk factors for AIDS—homosexual activity and IV drug use—are highly stigmatized in the U.S. Many people are unable or unwilling to admit their risk activities because of this.

"I know a doctor who says he/she thinks AIDS might be casually transmitted."

AIDS research is a highly specialized field, and most physicians are not AIDS specialists. They have to interpret what they hear and read just as non- physicians do. In a 1986 survey by MD magazine, 34% of private practice physicians responding believed food handlers should be tested for AIDS antibodies, presumably because they were concerned about the possibility of casual transmission.

This does not mean that there is a preponderance of scientific opinion favoring casual transmission. It means physicians, like everyone else, need careful and thorough education about AIDS risks. If you surveyed AIDS specialists who work with AIDS patients every day, you would find that they are quite confident that AIDS is not casually transmitted. You would see them following standard infection control guidelines to protect themselves from needle sticks or prolonged unprotected exposure to blood, vomitus, urine or feces. You would also see them touch their patients, talk with them, and sometimes laugh and cry with them. These caregivers know that as long as the standard guidelines about blood and wastes are followed, there is no need for artificial barriers to human caring and understanding.

We understand that doubts about casual transmission will continue for some people. Given the serious nature of the disease, this is understandable. We think a look at the scientific evidence shows very persuasively that AIDS is not transmitted without the intimate exchange of blood, semen, vaginal secretions or waste products. In all cases reported thus far, there is *no* case that has been shown to be transmitted through saliva, sweat, tears or any casual contact. If you personally continue to question the transmission of AIDS, we encourage you to ask further questions of AIDS information resources (see p. 153).

The Issue of Abstinence

We have heard a lot more talk about sexual abstinence since AIDS was first identified. Many people believe that teaching about abstinence is the best course for preventing the sexual transmission of AIDS among teenagers. There has been controversy about the issue, however, which we would like to address.

We couldn't agree more on the benefits of abstinence for teenagers. If more teens were abstinent, we would see fewer sexually transmitted diseases with their associated health problems (for example, pelvic inflammatory disease—PID—causes thousands of young women a year to become infertile). The rate of teenage pregnancy would also drop, and fewer young people would have to face the double burden of trying to complete their education while parenting a newborn or young child. And finally, we could expect the rate of AIDS infection to stay low in this age group. These are wonderful benefits, so promoting abstinence certainly has its place in teen education.

The problem arises when people suggest that abstinence is the *only* acceptable teaching for AIDS prevention. Adolescents are making their own decisions about sexual behavior, whether we want them to or not. American adolescents today are deciding in significant numbers not to be sexually abstinent. If we present abstinence as the only method of AIDS prevention, we are offering nothing to the twelve million teenagers in this country who are sexually active. We are essentially saying to them, "Be abstinent or die."

If we want to promote abstinence among teenagers, we must devote time, energy and effort to the task. Teens are surrounded by overt and covert messages from peers, in young adult fiction, in movies, television and advertising, and in popular music that endorse and encourage sexual activity. There are few resources in popular culture that suggest abstinence is a positive or desirable choice. To help teens balance the picture, we can teach them skills related to values clarification, decision making and assertiveness. To help them resist these compelling persuasions to be sexually active, we must promote teen self-esteem. These lessons are well beyond the scope of AIDS education alone. Careful planning of curricula in family life education and modern living skills, spanning the full course of a student's school career, can establish the foundation needed to develop such capabilities.

In providing teens a thorough and careful education about AIDS, we want to emphasize that abstinence is the only 100% effective method of preventing the sexual transmission of the AIDS virus. By also including a description of safer sex activities, we acknowledge that sexual activity does or might take place, now or in the future. We are not promoting teen sexual activity in these programs, however, and we can state this clearly to our students. What we are endorsing is care and thoughtfulness about decisions that affect oneself and one's friends or sexual partners. What we are supporting is health and longevity. What we hope to prevent is unnecessary suffering and death.

Teens (and adults) *deserve* full information about AIDS prevention. If we offer them less, we lose credibility as educators and as role models. If, in our AIDS education efforts, we neglect to acknowledge teenagers as people who may be sexually active, we lose a valuable opportunity to stem the spread of this devastating illness. If we fail to encourage those who are, or may someday be, sexually active to consider their choices carefully and reevaluate past decisions, we condemn them to a risk they might not otherwise choose to take.

We cannot afford to make these errors. The lives of our youth, of the adults they will become, and the children they will bear are much too precious. In our education efforts, we can present abstinence as the best of several possible choices for teens, but we must be honest and forthright about the full spectrum of prevention options for a population already quite active sexually.

Trouble-Shooting for Teachers: What Can Go Wrong in Teaching About AIDS?

AIDS is an interesting topic, and one that is relevant to young adults. Most classes in our experience have responded in an enthusiastic and appropriate manner to our presentations. Occasional difficulties might arise, so we share our suggestions for these situations.

1.   **Students do not respond to the materials.**

Many causes may underlie a lack of participation (including the other points listed below). If poor participation is atypical of a class, we suggest asking directly what the hesitation is about, or addressing the issues below. If the class continues to be unresponsive, carefully review AIDS transmission and prevention information in a lecture format, and use a worksheet or the test as an in-class tool.

2.   **Students are anxious about the sexual aspects of the material.**

Anxiety may manifest by withdrawal (silence) or acting out (disruption). Several issues about sexuality may arise.

Many people, including teenagers, associate AIDS with homosexuality. Where there is significant underlying homophobia—fear of or discomfort with homosexuality—AIDS education can be difficult. Addressing students' feelings about homosexuality may be appropriate in this instance. It is *essential* to clarify AIDS is not solely a disease of gay men.

Students may not be accustomed to discussing sex frankly with an older adult. They may be affected by new information about human sexual practices (especially oral and anal sex). Since adolescence is a time of social and sexual maturation, many students are only beginning to consider their feelings about sexuality. Their uncertainty about their own and their peers' attitudes may create further anxiety. If students are sexually active themselves, they may be concerned that this information will be revealed against their wishes (by other students in the class; by saying something unintentionally themselves; by some magical omniscience on the part of the teacher; etc.). If the students perceive that the teacher is uncomfortable with the material, they may try to "protect" the teacher by avoiding the lesson. In any of these instances, or others that might arise, talking about the situation directly and matter-of-factly usually helps lower anxiety.

3. **Students do not seem to understand the information.**

Some of the units in this curriculum are sophisticated and difficult. Select materials carefully and gear the academic demands of the lesson to the capabilities of the class. Too simple a presentation may bore students; too complex a class will lose them.

4. **The teacher does not know the answers to some questions**

This is to be expected and is not really a problem. You might write down unanswered questions, get the answers from information resources (see p. 153) and report back to the class; or use Worksheet 4: "Finding Answers to Questions About AIDS" (p. 111).

5. **Parents disapprove of the materials.**

We urge you to follow the guidelines of your school or district in seeking parental approval for teaching these materials. We believe the reasons for teaching youth about AIDS are *very* persuasive (as outlined in "Why Teach Teenagers and Young Adults About AIDS?," p.1). But we acknowledge not all parents will agree.

School districts and AIDS organizations can help with this problem by providing educational programs for parents.

Talking About Sexuality in Classrooms

Effective teaching about AIDS requires frank talk about sexuality. For teachers of subjects in which sex may not normally be a focus (science, social studies, etc.), this might raise some concerns. Though the usual techniques of good teaching do not change, a few guidelines can help in any class of young (or old) adults when talking about sexuality. We offer the following suggestions:

1. Personal boundaries need to be respected. No one should be asked to disclose opinions about sexuality if they do not wish to do so. Neither teacher nor students are expected to reveal personal experiences in these classes.

2. Each person has his or her own personal values about sexuality, and these will not be the same for everyone in the class. Differences are acknowledged and accepted. People are not put down for their values.

3. In discussions, it is necessary to clarify the difference between statements of fact ("It is true that...") and personal opinion ("I believe that..."). The teacher may occasionally need to assist students with such clarifications.

4. We recommend confidentiality rules be established for the class. This means personal opinions, values and experiences shared in the class are not discussed with others outside of the class. The teacher is also expected to maintain confidentiality, except in an instance where something illegal or dangerous (such as sexual abuse) is disclosed in class.

5. Anyone, including the teacher, may be embarrassed by questions or discussions about certain aspects of sexuality. This is normal, expected and acceptable.

6. Any question is reasonable. The teacher will not know all the answers. The teacher and class together can figure out how to find out about unanswered questions.

7. If any students have complaints about the topic, the method of teaching, or other aspects of the class, they are encouraged to discuss this directly with the teacher.

How to Teach About Condom Use

As more educators look to the task of providing AIDS education to teens, more may find themselves in a circumstance where instructions for using condoms are included in the lesson.

We recommend the following general guidelines for teaching about condom use:

1.   Be familiar with how condoms are used.

2.   Be familiar with different approaches to teaching condom use. In teaching, select an approach that will be comfortable for you and appropriate for your students.

3.   Be familiar with established guidelines in your school or community for teaching this material. Select teaching approaches appropriately.

To help you follow these guidelines, we expand on the first two points below.

HOW CONDOMS ARE USED

General instructions for condom use can be given briefly and simply. We have included quite a bit of detail here to cover most questions which are likely to arise about condom use.

We recommend latex condoms for disease prevention—natural skin condoms are not as effective in preventing the transmission of the AIDS virus. Condoms are not *100%* effective in preventing AIDS, but when properly and consistently used they are probably at least 98% effective. Sexual abstinence is the only 100% effective method for preventing the sexual transmission of AIDS.

1.   Use a condom every time you have intercourse, for all types of intercourse (oral, vaginal, anal). There is no "safe" period during which diseases are not transmitted.

2.   Keep condoms conveniently stored in a cool, dry place. If they are easy to get to, they will be easy to use. Do not keep them in a wallet or near direct heat or sunlight for long—the latex may weaken and the condom break during use.

3.   Open the package carefully, and handle the condoms gently. Jagged nails or rough handling can tear the condom.

4.   Do not test condoms by inflating or stretching them. The latex has been pretested

131

in a factory for its strength and ability to expand.

5.   As soon as erection occurs, put the condom on. First, with thumb and forefinger, gently press any air out of the receptacle tip at the closed end (air bubbles can cause condoms to break). If the condom is plain-ended, leave about a half inch free at the tip to catch the ejaculation. A dab of lubricant in the tip will solve the air problem *and* increase sensation.

6.   Use some lubrication on the outside of the condom and around the vagina or anus before entry. Use more as needed. *Use only water based lubricants* and read lubricant labels very carefully. Any lubricant containing fats, shortening or oils (such as Vaseline or cooking fats) will damage the latex and cause breakage.

        Lubricants or contraceptive jellies or foam containing a 5% or greater solution of the spermicide non-oxynol 9 offer additional protection against HIV infection.

7.   Hold the rim of the condom when necessary, including while withdrawing the penis, to keep the condom from slipping off. Withdraw gently.

8.   Throw used condoms away! Never use more than once.

9.   Using condoms may be difficult or embarrassing at first. This becomes easier, more natural and more relaxed when you are familiar with condom use.

WAYS TO TEACH ABOUT CONDOM USE

In any instruction about condom use, certain approaches are suggested. Many educators of adolescents prefer to use the passive rather than the active voice in discussing condom use ("Condoms should be used every time a person has intercourse," rather than "Use condoms every time you have intercourse,") because it is less likely to be interpreted as an endorsement or encouragement of teen sexual activity. Be as explicit as you reasonably can given your setting and your own comfort with the material. Having condoms for students to touch and examine helps demystify the whole process of condom use. If this is not practical, having one to show the class is useful. Be sure to have referral sources listed for students as to where they can acquire condoms and lubricants, how much they cost, and where they can get further questions answered.

1.   **Verbal instruction**: You can describe condoms and how they are used. Students will need to know basic vocabulary and physiology, so they are familiar with terms like "erection," "base of penis," and so forth.

2.   **Written instructions**: As an adjunct to lessons on condom use, you can hand out brochures showing how condoms are used. These are usually available from condom manufacturers or distributors, or from health clinics.

3.   **Visual instruction**: Describing how condoms are used, with visual aids to assist

the introduction, offers the most effective approach to condom education. Be sure to practice any method before trying it out in front of a group of students, so you are quite familiar with how sturdy condoms are when properly handled. Most simply, one can unwrap a condom and unroll it over the index and middle finger of one hand, showing how much space to leave at the tip, how to hold the end of the condom, and how to unroll and remove the condom. Some teachers are able to combine humor with demonstration by bringing cucumbers or zucchini to class and showing how to apply and remove condoms.

Expect humor, laughter and embarrassment in condom lessons. This is healthy! It shows that the message is getting through. Allowing students to address their embarrassment in class makes it less essential that they hide their feelings in real-life circumstances where honesty and frankness about condoms is essential.

Instructions for Cleaning Needles

The *best* strategy for preventing transmission of AIDS through needle use is not to use needles!

If you do use needles, the only sure way of avoiding AIDS is never to share.

Cleaning needles with bleach will kill AIDS virus in used needles. This is how it is done:

1. Pour liquid bleach into a glass.
    Fill the syringe with bleach.
    Empty bleach from syringe into a sink.
    Repeat.

2. Fill a glass with clean water.
    Fill the syringe with water.
    Empty water from the syringe into a sink.
    Repeat.

You must follow both steps. Make sure you don't shoot or drink the bleach. Throw away used bleach.

Staying Updated on AIDS Information

The changes in our knowledge about AIDS have been truly remarkable. In 1981, when the disease was first recognized and described, we did not even have a clue to its cause. Today (1987), we understand transmission, the causative virus has been identified, we know how to prevent the disease, and a successful antibody test has been developed.

Information about AIDS will continue to change. This certainly brings up the question of how up-to-date the materials in this curriculum will be in a short time. Briefly, here are the likely changes we will see in AIDS in the next few years:

1. **Epidemiology**: The number of cases will continue to increase dramatically. The U.S. Public Health Service predicts 270,000 total cases by 1991. Gay and bisexual men will continue to be the major group affected, but the overall percentage of cases among gay men will drop. IV drug users will be diagnosed in increasing numbers. Sexual transmission among heterosexuals will also increase, though most experts do not expect the disease to infect the heterosexual population as widely as it has gay men.

2. **Transmission**: Our knowledge about the transmission of AIDS will not change in any significant way. Exchange of blood, semen, vaginal secretions (and urine or feces) in sexual activities will be the primary mode of transmission, with sharing of needles in IV drug use a significant infection risk as well.

3. **Vaccine**: It is unlikely a successful vaccine will be developed soon, but work continues in this area. Once a vaccine is identified, several years of testing will be necessary before it is widely available.

4. **Treatment**: New treatment therapies are always under investigation. In 1987, a drug called AZT (Retrovir) has been used for people with HIV infection. It is the first federally approved drug which has shown a positive effect for persons with AIDS. AZT does not cure the immune system defect, but it does prolong life. Unfortunately, the side effects are so severe that about 50% of those who try to use the drug will be unable to do so. Further drugs will be developed and tested in the future, hopefully with greater benefits and fewer side effects. An actual cure is almost certainly much farther away.

5. **Antibody testing**: We may see the appearance of an inexpensive test that detects the presence of the virus rather than the antibody. Such a test, if it is reliable, could improve the accuracy of screening and diagnostic efforts. Antibody testing might become obsolete in this circumstance.

The basic information about AIDS—that it is a very serious disease that can be spread by sexual contact and the sharing of needles in IV drug use; that it is not casually transmitted; that it can be prevented; and that people need clear and accurate information about AIDS prevention—will not change.

Major changes in information about AIDS as well as updates on the number of cases reported are often reported in newspapers and news magazines. If you have a local AIDS organization, you can seek updates on information there. There is a list of resources on page 153 which can also provide you with current information about AIDS.

These guidelines reflect good basic hygiene. Most of the precautions are suggested primarily to protect the individual with HIV infection from exposure to disease, rather than to prevent transmission of the AIDS virus.

Infection Precautions for People with AIDS Living in the Community

By
Grace Lusby, MS, RN
Infection Control Coordinator,
San Francisco General Hospital

Helen Schietinger, MA, RN
Director,
Shanti AIDS Residence Program

San Francisco General Hospital Medical Special Care Unit and
San Francisco Bay Area Association for Practitioners of
Infection Control AIDS Resource Group

People with diagnosed AIDS who are able to care for themselves at home can safely live with both healthy individuals who do not have AIDS or with other persons with AIDS. Certain common sense hygienic measures protect both the person with AIDS as well as their housemates.

1.   Care should be taken to not share body secretions, particularly blood, semen or vaginal secretions, in sexual activities. This is important both to prevent possible transmission of AIDS to others and also to prevent acquiring other infections which may not be well tolerated by the person with AIDS.

       There is no reason why persons with AIDS should not continue to have the usual casual social contacts with people that they have had in the past.

2.   Maintaining a state of personal cleanliness is helpful to both the person with AIDS and others. This includes bathing regularly, washing hands after the use of bathroom facilities or contact with one's own body fluids such as semen, mucus, or blood, and washing hands before preparing food.

3.   Kitchen and bathroom facilities may be shared with others. Normal sanitary practices in any household will prevent the growth of fungi and bacteria that may potentially cause illness to both immunocompromised and immunocompetent people. These include:

a.　Clean kitchen counters with scouring powder to remove food particles. Sponges used to clean in the kitchen where food is prepared should NOT be the same sponges used to clean up bathroom-type spills. Dirty looking sponges should not be used to wash dishes or clean food preparation areas.

b.　Clean inside of refrigerator with soap and water to control molds.

c.　Mop kitchen floor at least once a week and clean up spills as they occur.

d.　Mop bathroom floor at least weekly and clean up spills. Bleach, 1:10 strength (1 part to 9 parts water) can be used to disinfect floor and shower floor (athletes foot is caused by a fungus which bleach will kill). 1:10 bleach can also be used in the sink. A little full strength bleach can be poured into the toilet bowl for disinfection. Any spills of body fluids or waste (blood, urine, stool, vomitus, etc.) should be cleaned up first and then the surface disinfected with 1:10 bleach.

e.　Sponges used to clean the floor or any body fluid spills SHOULD *NOT* BE USED TO WASH DISHES OR CLEAN FOOD PREPARATION AREAS. Mop water should NOT be poured down sink where food is prepared. Sponges used to clean up spills should not be washed out at sinks where food preparation occurs. Sponges and mops can be disinfected by soaking in 1:10 bleach for 5 minutes (longer may disintegrate sponge).

People with AIDS who are able to handle their own body secretions and excretions are able to live at home without any special precautions. Those listed above are considered good hygiene for any household.

4.　Dishes may be shared with others provided they are washed in soapy water hot enough to require gloves. A disinfectant does not need to be used.

5.　People with AIDS can safely cook for others provided they wash their hands before beginning. It's also a good idea not to lick the fingers or taste from the mixing spoon while cooking. (Advice for everyone.)

6.　Since unpasteurized milk and milk products have been associated with Salmonella infections in the past, these should not be included in the diet. Salmonella infections are not well tolerated by people with AIDS.

7.　If organically grown food is used (composted with human or animal feces), food should be cooked or peeled. "Organic" lettuce is not safe.

8.　Towels and wash cloths should not be shared without laundering. Toothbrushes, razors, enema equipment and sexual toys should not be shared.

9.　Trash disposal should be the same as for any household. Body wastes are flushed down the toilet. Other trash may be adequately handled by normal means (weekly trash pickups from cans lined with a plastic bag and a tight fitting lid to keep out rodents). In the event of large amounts of sputum, wound drainage, etc. on kleenex or dressings, it is a good idea to collect them in a lined trash can in the house.

10.   Pets — gloves should be used when cleaning bird cages (Psittacosis) and cat litter boxes (Toxoplasmosis). Tropical fish tanks may contain organisms in the Mycobacterium family which are not well tolerated by persons with AIDS. Get someone else to clean your tank.

11.   Keep living quarters well ventilated. Airborne diseases are less likely to be a problem when diluted by lots of air.

12.   Persons with AIDS can safely live together by observing the same common sense hygiene practices discussed above. The opportunistic infections acquired by persons with AIDS are caused by organisms commonly found in the environment. The risk of becoming sick from one of these infections is based on the amount of immune system impairment, not of casual household contact.

How Health Care Workers Can Protect Themselves from Infection on the Job

The guidelines for health care workers listed below are recommended for all patient contact and will protect one from exposure to the AIDS virus as well as most other diseases.

1.   Dispose of needles and syringes in puncture resistant containers without breaking or recapping the needle. Always dispose of needles immediately after use. Do not throw needles into regular trash.

2.   Wear gloves for contact with blood or body substances.

3.   Wear gloves or finger cot to cover a cut, abrasion, ulcer, rash or skin infection on your hands while working.

4.   Wash your hands as soon as possible after contact with blood or body substances or after touching objects which have been in contact with blood or body substances.

5.   Wear protective eye-wear when you are doing procedures which may result in splashes to the face (e.g., operative procedures, deliveries and endoscopies).

6.   Wear a mask when the patient is coughing and the diagnosis of tuberculosis has not been excluded or when performing a procedure which may result in splashes of blood or body fluids to the face and mucous membranes. Wear a mask when specified for communicable diseases which require respiratory precautions.

7.   Wear a gown when you expect spills of blood or body fluids onto your uniform or clothing or when contacting wounds or infected sites.

Infection Control Guidelines for Lab Classes Working with Body Fluids

✔ Review guidelines in the class before any work with body fluids is begun.

✔ Infection control guidelines will help prevent the transmission of many diseases, including hepatitis-B and HIV-infection (AIDS).

✔ Follow these guidelines at all times.

1. At the pre-college level, student work with human body fluids should be voluntary, with alternate lessons available for students who choose not to do such work.

2. Have students work only with their own body fluids (for blood typing or urinalysis, for example). Students with known blood-borne infections should not participate in such work.

3. Wear disposable latex gloves for all lab work involving human body fluids. Do not re-use gloves.

4. Use disposable needles and discard properly after use. Needles should not be re-capped or broken. Dispose of needles in puncture-resistant containers. Do not discard needles into regular trash.

5. Some lab work may involve the use of knives or scalpels (for example, for animal dissection). Train students in the proper use of such tools so that accidents where the skin might be cut or broken are avoided. If any tool has cut human skin or had other possible human blood exposure, discard it or sterilize it in a 1:10 solution of bleach. Similarly discard or sterilize any other lab equipment exposed to human blood.

6. *Never* use mouth suction with pipettes.

7. Spills of human body fluids, in or out of lab classes, should be cleaned by someone wearing disposable latex gloves. Wash the area with a 1:10 solution of bleach. Paper towels or rags used in clean-up may be wrapped in plastic bags and disposed of in regular trash. Mops should be well-rinsed in 1:10 bleach solution after the spill is cleaned.

8. Wear goggles for any lab work which might involve splashes of blood on the face or eyes.

9. Wash hands well with soap and hot water before and after any lab work. Wash any skin which has had contact with body fluids immediately with soap and water.

10. The atmosphere in lab classes should be such that students feel free to ask questions about infection control guidelines; are comfortable reporting any accidents exposing instruments to human blood; and adhere willingly, confidently and consistently to the guidelines.

CDC Classification System
for HIV Infections

(Adapted from *Morbidity and Mortality Weekly Report* 35 [May 23, 1986]: 334- 339.)

The classification system presented in this report is primarily applicable to public health purposes, including disease reporting and surveillance, epidemiologic studies, prevention and control activities, and public health policy and planning.

This system classifies the manifestations of HIV infection into four mutually exclusive groups. The classification system applies only to patients diagnosed as having HIV infection. Classification in a particular group is not explicitly intended to have prognostic significance, nor to designate severity of illness. However, classification in the four principal groups is hierarchical in that persons classified in a particular group should not be reclassified into a preceding group if clinical findings resolve, since clinical improvement may not accurately reflect changes in the severity of the underlying disease.

Group I. Acute HIV Infection.
A mononucleosis-like syndrome, characterized by high fevers, lymphadenopathy and rash, with or without aseptic meningitis, associated with seroconversion for HIV antibody. This illness usually lasts 10-14 days and appears two to eight weeks after initial infection with HIV. Not all persons infected will experience this illness.

Group II. Asymptomatic HIV Infection.
Absence of signs or symptoms of HIV infection. This is the category for asymptomatic carriers.

Group III. Persistent Generalized Lymphadenopathy (PGL).
The presence of palpable lymph node enlargement at two or more extrainguinal sites, persisting for more than 3 months in the absence of concurrent illness or condition other than HIV infection to explain the findings.

Group IV. Other HIV Disease.
The clinical manifestations of patients in this group may be designated by assignment to one or more subgroups (A-E) listed below. Any of these subgroups may include patients who are minimally symptomatic as well as those who are severely ill.

> **Subgroup A. Constitutional disease.**
> One or more of the following: fever persisting more than 1 month, involuntary weight loss of greater than 10% of baseline, or diarrhea persisting more than 1 month; and the absence of a concurrent illness or condition other than HIV infection to explain the findings.

Subgroup B. Neurologic disease.
One or more of the following: dementia, myelopathy, or peripheral neuropathy; and the absence of a concurrent illness or condition other than HIV infection to explain the findings.

Subgroup C. Secondary infection disease.
The diagnosis of an infection disease associated with HIV infection and/or at least moderately indicative of a defect in cell-mediated immunity. Divided further into two categories:

Category C-1.
Symptomatic or invasive disease due to one of 12 specified secondary infectious diseases listed in the surveillance definition of AIDS (see p. 149 for the full CDC definition of AIDS).

Category C-2.
Symptomatic or invasive disease due to one of 6 other specified secondary infectious diseases: oral hairy leukoplakia, multidermatomal herpes zoster, recurrent Salmonella bacteremia, nocardiosis, tuberculosis, or oral candidiasis (thrush).

Subgroup D. Secondary cancers.
Diagnosis of one or more kinds of cancer known to be associated with HIV infection as listed in the surveillance definition of AIDS (see p. 149) and at least moderatively indicative of a defect in cell-mediated immunity.

Subgroup E. Other conditions in HIV infection.
Other clinical findings or diseases, not classifiable above, that may be attributed to HIV infection and/or may be indicative of a defect in cell-mediated immunity.

*Group IV, Subgroup C, Category C-2, describes most persons with AIDS-related complex (ARC). Remember that the presence of tuberculosis, thrush or herpes zoster (shingles) without other evidence of HIV infection is not diagnostic of ARC, and that there are many people who may develop these illnesses for other reasons.

CDC
Case Definition for Acquired Immune Deficiency Syndrome

At its simplest, AIDS can be defined as the presence of either Pneumocystis carinii pneumonia (PCP), Kaposi's sarcoma (KS) (in a person less than 60 years of age), or other opportunistic infection, without any known underlying cause of immune suppression other than HIV infection. Earlier on, the list of opportunistic infections associated with an AIDS diagnosis was fairly short, but as knowledge of the disease grew, so did the number of opportunistic infections considered diagnostic of AIDS.

Today's CDC case definition of AIDS is considerably more complex than the one first issued in 1981. This is true for two main reasons: first, we have greater knowledge about the manifestations of serious HIV infection; second, laboratory measures have been developed to indicate the presence of HIV infection. For the full text of the current case definition, see *Morbidity and Mortality Weekly Report 36 Supplement* (August 14, 1987): 3S-15S. This definition is summarized and generalized here for those interested in this more technical information.

A person is considered to have a diagnosis of AIDS if he or she (1) has no known underlying cause of cellular immunodeficiency other than HIV infection; and (2) one or more of the following diseases has been definitively diagnosed. These conditions meet diagnostic criteria even if laboratory tests verifying HIV infection have not been performed.

1. Candidiasis of the esophagus, trachea, bronchi, or lungs

2. Cryptococcosis, extrapulmonary

3. Cryptosporidiosis with diarrhea persisting more than 1 month

4. Cytomegalovirus disease of an organ other than liver, spleen, or lymph nodes in a patient more than 1 month of age

5. Herpes simplex virus infection causing a mucocutaneous ulcer that persists longer than 1 month; or bronchitis, pneumonitis, or esophagitis for any duration affecting a patient more than 1 month of age

6. Kaposi's sarcoma affecting a patient less than 60 years of age

7. Lymphoma of the brain (primary) affecting a patient less than 60 years of age.

8. Lymphoid interstitial pneumonia and/or pulmonary lymphoid hyperplasia (LIP/PLH complex) affecting a child less than 13 years of age

9. *Mycobacterium avium* complex or *M. kansasii* disease, disseminated (at a site other than or in addition to lungs, skin, or cervical or hilar lymph nodes)

10. *Pneumocystis carinii* pneumonia

11. Progressive multifocal leukoencephalopathy

12. Toxoplasmosis of the brain affecting a patient more than 1 month of age

If an individual does have laboratory evidence for HIV infection, even if he or she has other known cause of immune deficiency, a diagnosis of AIDS is met by (1) the definitive diagnosis of any of the diseases listed above; or (2) the definitive diagnosis of any of the diseases listed below.

1. Bacterial infections, multiple or recurrent (any combination of at least two within a 2-year period), of the following types affecting a child less than 13 years of age:

   Septicemia, pneumonia, meningitis, bone or joint infection, or abscess of an internal organ or body cavity (excluding otitis media or superficial skin or mucosal abscesses), caused by *Haemophilus, Streptococcus* (including pneumococcus), or other pyogenic bacteria

2. Coccidioidomycosis, disseminated (at a site other than or in addition to lungs or cervical or hilar lymph nodes)

3. HIV encephalopathy (also called "HIV dementia," "AIDS dementia," or "subacute encephalitis due to HIV")

4. Histoplasmosis, disseminated (at a site other than or in addition to lungs or cervical or hilar lymph nodes)

5. Isosporiasis with diarrhea persisting more than 1 month

6. Kaposi's sarcoma at any age

7. Lymphoma of the brain (primary) at any age

8. Other non-Hodgkin's lymphoma of B-cell or unknown immunologic phenotype and the following histologic types:

   a. Small noncleaved lymphoma (either Burkitt or non-Burkitt type)

   b. Immunoblastic sarcoma (equivalent to any of the following, although not necessarily all in combination: immunoblastic lymphoma, large-cell lymphoma, diffuse histiocytic lymphoma, diffuse undifferentiated lymphoma, or high-grade lymphoma)

NOTE: Lymphomas are not included here if they are of T-cell immunologic phenotype or their histologic type is not described or is described as "lymphocytic," "lymphoblastic," "small cleaved," or "plasmacytoid lymphocytic"

9.   Any mycobacterial disease caused by mycobacteria other than *M. tuberculosis*, disseminated (at a site other than or in addition to lungs, skin, or cervical or hilar lymph nodes)

10. Disease caused by *M. tuberculosis*, extrapulmonary (involving at least one site outside the lungs, regardless of whether there is concurrent pulmonary involvement)

11. *Salmonella* (nontyphoid) septicemia, recurrent

12. HIV wasting syndrome (emaciation, "slim disease")

If a person has laboratory evidence of HIV infection, an AIDS diagnosis is also given if any of the following diseases are diagnosed presumptively. (In many of these illnesses, definitive diagnosis is available only by invasive procedures. Presumptive diagnosis may be made if the patient's condition precludes the possibility of such diagnostic efforts, or if the treating physician is quite familiar with the clinical manifestations and feels the procedures for definitive diagnosis are not necessary.)

1.   Candidiasis of the esophagus

2.   Cytomegalovirus retinitis with loss of vision

3.   Kaposi's sarcoma

4.   Lymphoid interstitial pneumonia and/or pulmonary lymphoid hyperplasia (LIP/PLH complex) affecting a child less than 13 years of age

5.   Mycobacterial disease (acid-fast bacilli with species not identified by culture), disseminated (involving at least one site other than or in addition to lungs, skin, or cervical or hilar lymph nodes)

6.   *Pneumocystis carinii* pneumonia

7.   Toxoplasmosis of the brain affecting a patient more than 1 month of age

AIDS Information Sources

The network of AIDS information and service resources is large. There are organizations or agencies responsible for coordinating AIDS services in every state. The national information number, listed below, maintains up-to- date listings of local resources throughout the country. Not all of these organizations have information hotlines.

Be sure to check any numbers or addresses before giving them to students—they have a tendency to change fairly often.

HOTLINES

National AIDS Hotline
(800) 342-AIDS—Toll-free
(202) 245-6867—Collect from Alaska and Hawaii
Administered by the Social Health Association

National Gay Task Force
AIDS Information Hotline
(800) 221-7044
(212) 807-6016 (NY State)

STD National Hotline
(800) 227-8922
Administered by the American Social Health Association

WRITTEN RESOURCES: PAMPHLETS, BROCHURES, POSTERS

Call or write for description of materials and price list. Some of these agencies will also provide speakers for school assemblies, consultation for teachers or education for parents.

California

AIDS Project, Los Angeles
1362 Santa Monica Blvd.
Los Angeles, CA 90046
(213) 876-AIDS

Network Publications
A Division of ETR Associates
P.O. Box 1830
Santa Cruz, CA 95061-1830
(408) 438-4080

California (cont.)

San Francisco AIDS Foundation
333 Valencia St.
San Francisco, CA 94103
(415) 863-2437

Maryland

Health Education and Resource
Organization (HERO)
101 W. Read St., Suite 812
Baltimore, MD 21201
(301) 685-1180

Massachusetts

AIDS Action Committee
661 Boylston St.
Boston, MA 02116
(617) 536-7733

New York

Gay Men's Health Crisis, Inc.
132 W. 24th St.
New York, NY 10011
(212) 807-6655

Hispanic AIDS Forum
140 W. 22nd St., Suite 301
New York, NY 10011
(212) 463-8264

North Carolina

American Social Health Association
P.O. Box 13827
Research Triangle Park, NC 27709
(919) 361-2742

Washington, DC

American Red Cross
AIDS Education Office
1730 D St., N.W.
Washington, DC 20006
(202) 737-8300
or contact local Red Cross

National AIDS Network
1012 14th St. NW, Suite 601
Washington, D.C. 20005
(202) 347-0390

U.S. Public Health Service
Public Affairs Office
Hubert H. Humphrey Building
Room 725-H
200 Independence Ave., S.W.
Washington, DC 20201
(202) 245-6867

GLOSSARY

AIDS

Acquired Immune Deficiency Syndrome. A viral disease which damages the body's immune system, making the infected person susceptible to a wide range of serious diseases. May also involve neurologic symptoms.

antibody

Proteins produced in the blood in response to toxins or other foreign organisms. Antibodies in some cases can neutralize toxins and help eliminate infections, though in the case of AIDS, antibodies are not effective in combating the disease.

ARC

AIDS-related complex. A diagnosis given to people infected with the AIDS virus who have symptoms of illness related to this infection, but do not meet the diagnostic criteria necessary to be given a diagnosis of AIDS.

ARV

The name given the AIDS virus by Jay Levy of the University of California, San Francisco. Stands for AIDS-associated retrovirus.

blood transfusion

To put blood into the veins of an individual. First, blood is withdrawn from a donor. It may be stored for some period of time. Then, to treat injury or illness, a recipient is given this donated blood.

casual contact

Normal day-to-day contact between people at home, school, work or in the community, which does not involve sexual interactions or the sharing of needles.

casual transmission

Transmission of disease through casual contact. Colds and flus are often casually transmitted. The AIDS virus is not transmitted casually.

CDC

The Centers for Disease Control, a federal agency based in Atlanta which studies and monitors the incidence and prevalence of disease in the U.S., and also provides health and safety guidelines for the prevention of disease.

condoms

Also called rubbers or prophylactics. A latex sheath used to cover the penis during intercourse to prevent pregnancy and the transmission of sexual diseases. Latex

155

condoms are effective in preventing the transmission of the AIDS virus. "Natural skin" condoms are not as reliable for the prevention of disease.

disease

A particular destructive process in an organ or organism with a specific cause and characteristic symptoms; an illness.

ELISA

A test used to detect HIV antibodies in blood samples. The most inexpensive and widely used test to date. Stands for enzyme-linked immunosorbent assay.

epidemiology

The study of the distribution and causes of diseases.

false negative

In an AIDS antibody test, a result that reads negative when there is actually antibody in the blood. A type of erroneous result.

false positive

In an AIDS antibody test, a result that reads positive when there is actually no antibody in the blood. A type of erroneous result.

hemophilia

A rare, inherited bleeding disorder of males in which normal blood clotting is not possible. Treated with Factor VIII, a product made of human blood which allows normal clotting to occur.

HIV

The accepted scientific name for the AIDS virus, in most common usage now. Stands for human immunodeficiency virus.

HTLV-III

The name given the AIDS virus by Robert Gallo of the National Cancer Institute. Stands for human T-cell lymphotropic virus, type three.

IFA

A test used to detect HIV antibodies in blood samples. More difficult to perform and more expensive than the ELISA. Also believed to be more specific (can accurately identify samples without antibody) than the ELISA, so sometimes used to verify ELISA results. Stands for immunofluorescent assay.

immune system

The body's system of defense against disease, consisting of specialized cells and proteins in the blood and other body fluids.

incubation

In a medical context, the length of time between an individual first being infected with a disease-causing organism and the development of symptoms or diagnosis. The incubation period for AIDS averages over five years.

intercourse

A type of sexual contact involving one of the following: (1) insertion of a man's penis into a woman's vagina, called "vaginal intercourse"; (2) placement of the mouth on the genitals of another person, called "oral intercourse"; or (3) insertion of a man's penis into the anus of another person, called "anal intercourse."

intravenous

"Within veins"; injection by needles directly into the blood veins.

Kaposi's sarcoma

KS, a cancer or tumor of the blood and/or lymphatic vessel walls, sometimes seen in persons with AIDS. Usually appears as pink or purple blotches on the skin.

LAV

The name given the AIDS virus by Luc Montagnier of the Institute Pasteur, Paris. Stands for lymphadenopathy associated virus.

lubricant

In this context, a substance applied to condoms or sexual organs which makes contact between condom and skin slippery. Lubricated condoms are more comfortable, safe and exciting. Lubricants can be purchased in most places where condoms are sold. Use only *water based* lubricants with condoms, and read labels carefully—any fats or oils will break down the latex and may cause the condom to tear.

lymphadenopathy

The condition of lymph nodes being swollen. Often a sign of infection or illness. People infected with the AIDS virus often have chronic lymphadenopathy.

neurologic

Pertaining to the nervous system or brain. Persons infected with the AIDS virus often develop neurologic infection with symptoms such as forgetfulness, confusion, perceptual problems, lack of coordination or loss of muscle control.

non-oxynol 9

A spermicide which has also been shown to kill the AIDS virus in laboratory studies. Available in some sexual lubricants which can be used with condoms, non-oxynol 9 is *not* an effective AIDS prevention method used on its own. Concentrations of 5% or more are recommended.

opportunistic infection

An infection caused by organisms that are not able to affect people with healthy immune systems.

Pneumocystis carinii pneumonia

PCP, the most common life-threatening opportunistic illness diagnosed in AIDS. Caused by a protozoan parasite, it creates difficulty in breathing and is the most common cause of death for people with AIDS.

PWA

Person with AIDS. Many people with AIDS prefer this term to others like "AIDS victim," or "AIDS patient." They would rather see themselves as active participants in their treatment and healing, not helpless victims who passively wait to die. They are whole and complete persons, and the term "patient" reduces them to little more than a case of disease.

risk

The chance of injury, damage or loss; dangerous chance; hazard.

safer sex

Sexual activity which protects one from infection with the AIDS virus. In safer sex, no body fluids are shared.

secretion

A substance generated from blood or cells which may have cleansing, lubricating or other characteristics.

seropositive

In the case of AIDS, the condition of having AIDS virus antibodies found in the blood.

spermicide

Any substance used to help prevent pregnancy because of its ability to kill sperm. One spermicide, non-oxynol 9, has also been shown to kill the AIDS virus in laboratory studies.

STD

Sexually transmitted disease, any of a number of diseases which can be transmitted through various forms of sexual contact. AIDS is a disease which is transmitted through sexual intercourse.

surveillance

In public health terms, monitoring and collecting data on incidence of disease— essentially, counting the number of cases.

T-cell

A specialized white blood cell which helps orchestrate the immune system's response to infection. The T-cell is invaded and disabled by the HIV virus.

transmission

Passed along. In the context of disease, passed from one individual to another.

vaccine

A preparation introduced to the body to produce immunity to disease. Historically, most vaccines have been made of weakened, or killed disease organisms themselves. In the future, we may see vaccines which are genetically engineered non-lethal forms of such organisms.

virus

An organism formed of genes surrounded by a protein coating. Technically not living, since it cannot reproduce itself. Smaller than any living organism.

Western Blot

A test used to detect HIV antibodies in blood samples. More difficult to perform, and more expensive, than the ELISA. Also believed to be more specific (can accurately identify samples without antibody) than the ELISA, so sometimes used to verify ELISA results.